Virtual Clinical Excursions—Obstetrics

for

Lowdermilk and Perry:
Maternity Nursing
8th Edition

D1232902

Virtual Clinical Excursions—Obstetrics

for

Lowdermilk and Perry:
Maternity Nursing
8th Edition

prepared by

Kim D. Cooper, RN, MSN
Ivy Tech Community College
Terre Haute, Indiana

software developed by

Wolfsong Informatics, LLC
Tucson, Arizona

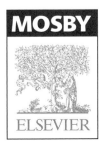

MOSBY

ELSEVIER

11830 Westline Industrial Dr.
St. Louis, Missouri 63146

VIRTUAL CLINICAL EXCURSIONS—OBSTETRICS FOR
LOWDERMILK AND PERRY:
MATERNITY NURSING
EIGHTH EDITION

ISBN: 978-0-323-07392-9

Copyright © 2011, 2007 by Mosby, Inc., an affiliate of Elsevier Inc.

Notice

Knowledge and best practice in this field are constantly changing. As new research and experience
broaden our knowledge, changes in practice, treatment and drug therapy may become necessary or
appropriate. Readers are advised to check the most current information provided (i) on procedures
featured or (ii) by the manufacturer of each product to be administered, to verify the recommended
dose or formula, the method and duration of administration, and contraindications. It is the
responsibility of the practitioner, relying on their own experience and knowledge of the patient, to
make diagnoses, to determine dosages and the best treatment for each individual patient, and to
take all appropriate safety precautions. To the fullest extent of the law, neither the Publisher nor
the Authors assumes any liability for any injury and/or damage to persons or property arising out
or related to any use of the material contained in this book.

ISBN: 978-0-323-07392-9

Executive Editor: *Tom Wilhelm*
Managing Editor: *Jeff Downing*
Associate Developmental Editor: *Krissy Prysmiki*
Project Manager: *Joy Moore*

Printed in the United States of America

Last digit is the print number: 9 8 7 6 5 4 3 2 1

Workbook prepared by

Kim D. Cooper, RN, MSN
Ivy Tech Community College
Terre Haute, Indiana

Previous edition prepared by

Kitty Cashion, RN, BC, MSN
Clinical Nurse Specialist
University of Tennessee Health Science Center
College of Medicine
Department of Obstetrics & Gynecology
Division of Maternal-Fetal Medicine
Memphis, Tennessee

Kelly Ann Crum, RN, MSN
Chair, Department of Nursing
Associate Professor of Nursing
Maranatha Baptist Bible College
Watertown, Wisconsin

Textbook

Deitra Leonard Lowdermilk, RNC, PhD, FAAN
Clinical Professor Emerita, School of Nursing
University of North Carolina at Chapel Hill
Chapel Hill, North Carolina

Shannon E. Perry, RN, CNS, PhD, FAAN
Professor Emerita, School of Nursing
San Francisco State University
San Francisco, California

Reviewer

Bella Smith, RN, MSN, CCRN
Nursing Education Consultant
B. Smith Associates
Tucson, Arizona

Contents

Table of Contents
Lowdermilk and Perry:
Maternity Nursing, 8th Edition

Getting Started

GETTING SET UP

■ **MINIMUM SYSTEM REQUIREMENTS**

WINDOWS®

Windows Vista™, XP, 2000 (Recommend Windows XP/2000)
Pentium® III processor (or equivalent) @ 600 MHz (Recommend 800 MHz or better)
256 MB of RAM (Recommend 1 GB or more for Windows Vista)
800 x 600 screen size (Recommend 1024 x 768)
Thousands of colors
12x CD-ROM drive
Soundblaster 16 soundcard compatibility
Stereo speakers or headphones

Note: Windows Vista and XP require administrator privileges for installation.

MACINTOSH®

MAC OS X (10.2 or higher)
Apple Power PC G3 @ 500 MHz or better
128 MB of RAM (Recommend 256 MB or more)
800 x 600 screen size (Recommend 1024 x 768)
Thousands of colors
12x CD-ROM drive
Stereo speakers or headphones

1

■ INSTALLATION INSTRUCTIONS

WINDOWS

1. Insert the *Virtual Clinical Excursions—Obstetrics* CD-ROM.
2. The setup screen should appear automatically if the current product is not already installed. Windows Vista users may be asked to authorize additional security prompts.
3. Follow the onscreen instructions during the setup process.

   If the setup screen does *not* appear automatically (and *Virtual Clinical Excursions—Obstetrics* has not been installed already):
   a. Click the **My Computer** icon on your desktop or on your Start menu.
   b. Double-click on your CD-ROM drive.
   c. If installation does not start at this point:
      (1) Click the **Start** icon on the taskbar and select the **Run** option.
      (2) Type d:\setup.exe (where "d:\" is your CD-ROM drive) and press **OK**.
      (3) Follow the onscreen instructions for installation.

MACINTOSH

1. Insert the *Virtual Clinical Excursions—Obstetrics* CD in the CD-ROM drive. The disk icon will appear on your desktop.

2. Double-click on the disk icon.

3. Double-click on the OBSTETRICS_MAC run file.

Note: Virtual Clinical Excursions—Obstetrics for Macintosh does not have an installation setup and can only be run directly from the CD.

■ HOW TO USE VIRTUAL CLINICAL EXCURSIONS—OBSTETRICS

WINDOWS

1. Double-click on the *Virtual Clinical Excursions—Obstetrics* icon located on your desktop.
2. Or navigate to the program via the Windows Start menu.

Note: If your computer uses Windows Vista, right-click on the desktop shortcut and choose **Properties**. In the Compatibility Mode, check the box for "Run as Administrator." Below is a screen capture to show what this looks like.

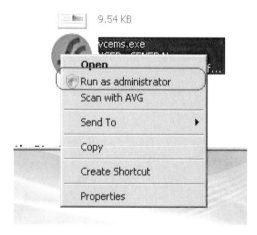

■ MACINTOSH

    1.   Insert the *Virtual Clinical Excursions—Obstetrics* CD in the CD-ROM drive. The disk icon will appear on your desktop.

    2.   Double-click on the disk icon.

    3.   Double-click on the OBSTETRICS_MAC run file.

SCREEN SETTINGS

For best results, your computer monitor resolution should be set at a minimum of 800 x 600. The number of colors displayed should be set to "thousands or higher" (High Color or 16 bit) or "millions of colors" (True Color or 24 bit).

Windows

1. From the **Start** menu, select **Control Panel** (on some systems, you will first go to **Settings**, then to **Control Panel**).
2. Double-click on the **Display** icon.
3. Click on the **Settings** tab.
4. Under **Screen resolution** use the slider bar to select **800 by 600 pixels**.
5. Access the **Colors** drop-down menu by clicking on the down arrow.
6. Select **High Color (16 bit)** or **True Color (24 bit)**.
7. Click on **OK**.
8. You may be asked to verify the setting changes. Click **Yes**.
9. You may be asked to restart your computer to accept the changes. Click **Yes**.

Macintosh

1. Select the **Monitors** control panel.
2. Select **800 x 600** (or similar) from the **Resolution** area.
3. Select **Thousands** or **Millions** from the **Color Depth** area.

■ WEB BROWSERS

Supported web browsers include Microsoft Internet Explorer (IE) version 6.0 or higher and Mozilla Firefox version 2.0 or higher. The supported browser for Macs running OS X is Mozilla Firefox.

If you use America Online® (AOL) for web access, you will need AOL version 4.0 or higher and one of the browsers listed above. Do not use earlier versions of AOL with earlier versions of IE, because you will have difficulty accessing many features.

For best results with AOL:
- Connect to the Internet using AOL version 4.0 or higher.
- Open a private chat within AOL (this allows the AOL client to remain open, without asking whether you wish to disconnect while minimized).
- Minimize AOL.
- Launch a recommended browser.

■ **TECHNICAL SUPPORT**

Technical support for this product is available between 7:30 a.m. and 7 p.m. (CST), Monday through Friday. Before calling, be sure that your computer meets the minimum system requirements to run this software. Inside the United States and Canada, call 1-800-692-9010. Outside North America, call 314-872-8370. You may also fax your questions to 314-523-4932 or contact Technical Support through e-mail: technical.support@elsevier.com.

Trademarks: Windows, Macintosh, Pentium, and America Online are registered trademarks.

Copyright © 2011, 2007 by Mosby, Inc., an affiliate of Elsevier Inc.

All rights reserved. No part of this product may be reproduced or transmitted in any form or by any means, electronic or mechanical, including input or storage in any information system, without written permission from the publisher.

ACCESSING *Virtual Clinical Excursions—Obstetrics* FROM EVOLVE

The product you have purchased is part of the Evolve family of online courses and learning resources. Please read the following information thoroughly to get started.

To access your instructor's course on Evolve:

Your instructor will provide you with the username and password needed to access this specific course on the Evolve Learning System. Once you have received this information, please follow these instructions:

1. Go to the Evolve student page (http://evolve.elsevier.com/student).

2. Enter your username and password in the **Login to My Evolve** area and click the **Login** button.

3. You will be taken to your personalized **My Evolve** page, where the course will be listed in the **My Courses** module.

TECHNICAL REQUIREMENTS

To use an Evolve course, you will need access to a computer that is connected to the Internet and equipped with web browser software that supports frames. For optimal performance, it is recommended that you have speakers and use a high-speed Internet connection. However, slower dial-up modems (56 K minimum) are acceptable.

Whichever browser you use, the browser preferences must be set to enable cookies and the cache must be set to reload every time.

Enable Cookies

Browser	Steps
Internet Explorer (IE) 6.0 or higher	1. Select **Tools** → **Internet Options**. 2. Select **Privacy** tab. 3. Use the slider (slide down) to **Accept All Cookies**. 4. Click **OK**. -OR- 3. Click the **Advanced** button. 4. Click the check box next to **Override Automatic Cookie Handling**. 5. Click the **Accept** radio buttons under **First-party Cookies** and **Third-party Cookies**. 6. Click **OK**.
Mozilla Firefox 2.0 or higher	1. Select **Tools** → **Options**. 2. Select the **Privacy** icon. 3. Click to expand Cookies. 4. Select **Allow sites to set cookies**. 5. Click **OK**.

Set Cache to Always Reload a Page

Browser	Steps
Internet Explorer (IE) 6.0 or higher	1. Select **Tools** → **Internet Options**. 2. Select **General** tab. 3. Go to the **Temporary Internet Files** and click the **Settings** button. 4. Select the radio button for **Every visit to the page** and click **OK** when complete.
Mozilla Firefox 2.0 or higher	1. Select **Tools** → **Options**. 2. Select the **Privacy** icon. 3. Click to expand Cache. 4. Set the value to "0" in the **Use up to:** __ **MB of disk space for the cache** field. 5. Click **OK**.

Plug-Ins

 Adobe Acrobat Reader—With the free Acrobat Reader software, you can view and print Adobe PDF files. Many Evolve products offer student and instructor manuals, checklists, and more in this format!

Download at: http://www.adobe.com

 Apple QuickTime—Install this to hear word pronunciations, heart and lung sounds, and many other helpful audio clips within Evolve Online Courses!

Download at: http://www.apple.com

 Adobe Flash Player—This player will enhance your viewing of many Evolve web pages, as well as educational short-form to long-form animation within the Evolve Learning System!

Download at: http://www.adobe.com

 Adobe Shockwave Player—Shockwave is best for viewing the many interactive learning activities within Evolve Online Courses!

Download at: http://www.adobe.com

 Microsoft Word Viewer—With this viewer, Microsoft Word users can share documents with those who don't have Word, and users without Word can open and view Word documents. Many Evolve products have testbank, student and instructor manuals, and other documents available for downloading and viewing on your own computer!

Download at: http://www.microsoft.com

 Microsoft PowerPoint Viewer—With this viewer, you can access PowerPoint 97, 2000, and 2002 presentations even if you don't have PowerPoint. Many Evolve products have slides available for downloading and viewing on your own computer!

Download at: http://www.microsoft.com

SUPPORT INFORMATION

Live phone support is available to customers in the United States and Canada at **800-401-9962** from 7:30 a.m. to 7 p.m. (CST), Monday through Friday. Support is also available through email at evolve-support@elsevier.com.

Online 24/7 support can be accessed on the Evolve website (http://evolve.elsevier.com). Resources include:

- Guided tours
- Tutorials
- Frequently asked questions (FAQs)
- Online copies of course user guides
- And much more!

A QUICK TOUR

Welcome to *Virtual Clinical Excursions—Obstetrics*, a virtual hospital setting in which you can work with multiple complex patient simulations and also learn to access and evaluate the information resources that are essential for high-quality patient care. The virtual hospital, Pacific View Regional Hospital, has realistic architecture and access to patient rooms, a Nurses' Station, and a Medication Room.

■ BEFORE YOU START

Make sure you have your textbook nearby when you use the *Virtual Clinical Excursions—Obstetrics* CD. You will want to consult topic areas in your textbook frequently while working with the CD and using this workbook.

■ HOW TO SIGN IN

- Enter your name on the Student Nurse identification badge.
- Now choose one of the four periods of care in which to work. In Periods of Care 1 through 3, you can actively engage in patient assessment, entry of data in the electronic patient record (EPR), and medication administration. Period of Care 4 presents the day in review. Click on the appropriate period of care. (For this quick tour, choose **Period of Care 1: 0730-0815**.)
- This takes you to the Patient List screen (see example on page 11). Note that the virtual time is provided in the box at the lower left corner of the screen (0730, since we chose Period of Care 1).

Note: If you choose to work during Period of Care 4: 1900-2000, the Patient List screen is skipped since you are not able to visit patients or administer medications during the shift. Instead, you are taken directly to the Nurses' Station, where the records of all the patients on the floor are available for your review.

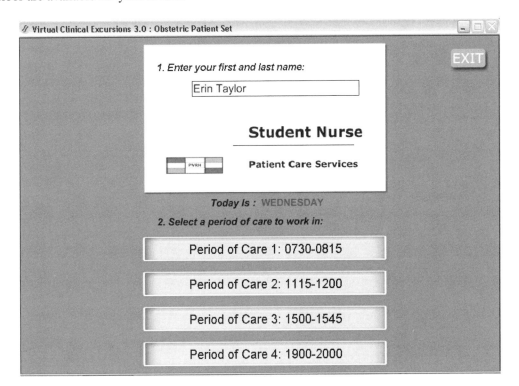

■ PATIENT LIST

OBSTETRICS UNIT

Dorothy Grant (Room 201)
30-week intrauterine pregnancy—A 25-year-old Caucasian multipara admitted with abdominal trauma following a domestic violence incident. Her complications include preterm labor and extensive social issues such as acquiring safe housing for her family upon discharge.

Stacey Crider (Room 202)
27-week intrauterine pregnancy—A 21-year-old Native American primigravida admitted for intravenous tocolysis, bacterial vaginosis, and poorly controlled insulin-dependent gestational diabetes. Strained family relationships and social isolation complicate this patient's ability to comply with strict dietary requirements and prenatal care.

Kelly Brady (Room 203)
26-week intrauterine pregnancy—A 35-year-old Caucasian primigravida urgently admitted for progressive symptoms of preeclampsia. A history of inadequate coping with major life stressors leave her at risk for a recurrence of depression as she faces a diagnosis of HELLP syndrome and the delivery of a severely premature infant.

Maggie Gardner (Room 204)
22-week intrauterine pregnancy—A 41-year-old African-American multigravida admitted for a high-risk pregnancy evaluation and rule out diagnosis of systemic lupus erythematosus. Coping with chronic pain, fatigue, and a history of multiple miscarriages contribute to an anxiety disorder and the need for social service intervention.

Gabriela Valenzuela (Room 205)
34-week intrauterine pregnancy—A 21-year-old Hispanic primigravida with a history of mitral valve prolapse admitted for uterine cramping and vaginal bleeding suggestive of placental abruption following an unrestrained motor vehicle accident. Her needs include staff support for an unprepared-for labor and possible preterm birth.

Laura Wilson (Room 206)
37-week intrauterine pregnancy—An 18-year-old Caucasian primigravida urgently admitted after being found unconscious at home. Her complications include HIV-positive status and chronic polysubstance abuse. Unrealistic expectations of parenthood and living with a chronic illness combined with strained family relations prompt comprehensive social and psychiatric evaluations initiated on the day of simulation.

■ HOW TO SELECT A PATIENT

- You can choose one or more patients to work with from the Patient List by checking the box to the left of the patient name(s). For this quick tour, select Dorothy Grant. (In order to receive a scorecard for a patient, the patient must be selected before proceeding to the Nurses' Station.)
- Click on **Get Report** to the right of the medical records number (MRN) to view a summary of the patient's care during the 12-hour period before your arrival on the unit.
- After reviewing the report, click on **Go to Nurses' Station** in the right lower corner to begin your care. (*Note:* If you have been assigned to care for multiple patients, you can click on **Return to Patient List** to select and review the report for each additional patient before going to the Nurses' Station.)

Note: Even though the Patient List is initially skipped when you sign in to work for Period of Care 4, you can still access this screen if you wish to review the shift report for any of the patients. To do so, simply click on **Patient List** near the top left corner of the Nurses' Station (or click on the clipboard to the left of the Kardex). Then click on **Get Report** for the patient(s) whose care you are reviewing. This may be done during any period of care.

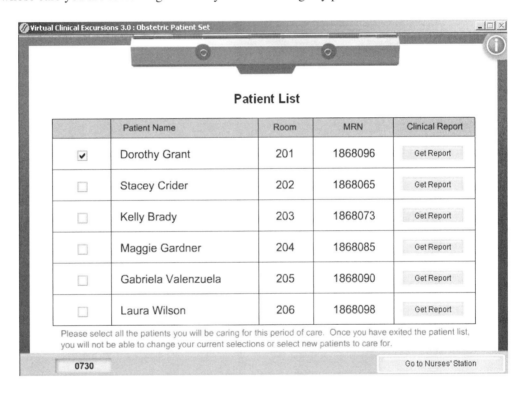

■ HOW TO FIND A PATIENT'S RECORDS

NURSES' STATION

Within the Nurses' Station, you will see:

1. A clipboard that contains the patient list for that floor.
2. A chart rack with patient charts labeled by room number, a notebook labeled Kardex, and a notebook labeled MAR (Medication Administration Record).
3. A desktop computer with access to the Electronic Patient Record (EPR).
4. A tool bar across the top of the screen that can also be used to access the Patient List, EPR, Chart, MAR, and Kardex. This tool bar is also accessible from each patient's room.
5. A Drug Guide containing information about the medications you are able to administer to your patients.
6. A tool bar across the bottom of the screen that can be used to access the Floor Map, patient rooms, Medication Room, and Drug Guide.

As you run your cursor over an item, it will be highlighted. To select, simply double-click on the item. As you use these resources, you will always be able to return to the Nurses' Station by clicking on the **Return to Nurses' Station** bar located in the right lower corner of your screen.

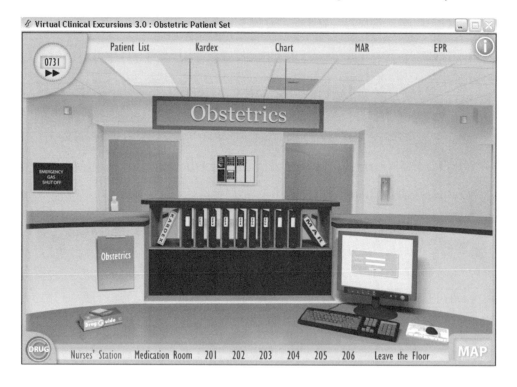

MEDICATION ADMINISTRATION RECORD (MAR)

The MAR icon located on the tool bar at the top of your screen accesses current 24-hour medications for each patient. Click on the icon and the MAR will open. (*Note:* You can also access the MAR by clicking on the MAR notebook on the far right side of the book rack in the center of the screen.) Within the MAR, tabs on the right side of the screen allow you to select patients by room number. Be careful to make sure you select the correct tab number for *your* patient rather than simply reading the first record that appears after the MAR opens. Each MAR sheet lists the following:

- Medications
- Route and dosage of each medication
- Times of administration of each medication

Note: The MAR changes each day. Expired MARs are stored in the patients' charts.

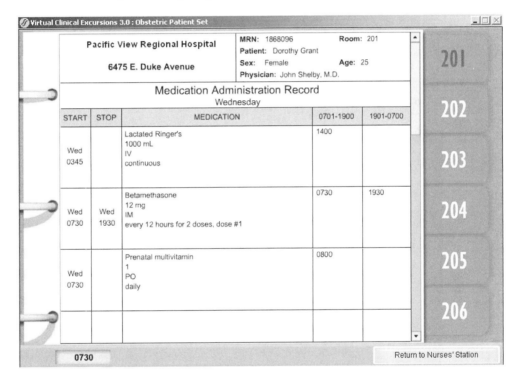

CHARTS

To access patient charts, either click on the **Chart** icon at the top of your screen or anywhere within the chart rack in the center of the Nurses' Station screen. When the close-up view appears, the individual charts are labeled by room number. To open a chart, click on the room number of the patient whose chart you wish to review. The patient's name and allergies will appear on the left side of the screen, along with a list of tabs on the right side of the screen, allowing you to view the following data:

- Allergies
- Physician's Orders
- Physician's Notes
- Nurse's Notes
- Laboratory Reports
- Diagnostic Reports
- Surgical Reports
- Consultations

- Patient Education
- History and Physical
- Nursing Admission
- Expired MARs
- Consents
- Mental Health
- Admissions
- Emergency Department

Information appears in real time. The entries are in reverse chronologic order, so use the down arrow at the right side of each chart page to scroll down to view previous entries. Flip from tab to tab to view multiple data fields or click on **Return to Nurses' Station** in the lower right corner of the screen to exit the chart.

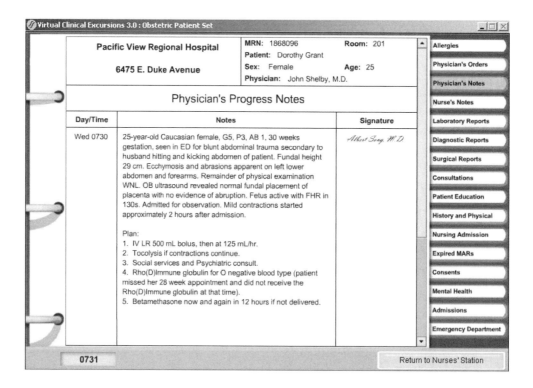

ELECTRONIC PATIENT RECORD (EPR)

The EPR can be accessed from the computer in the Nurses' Station or from the EPR icon located in the tool bar at the top of your screen. To access a patient's EPR:

- Click on either the computer screen or the **EPR** icon.
- Your username and password are automatically filled in.
- Click on **Login** to enter the EPR.
- *Note:* Like the MAR, the EPR is arranged numerically. Thus when you enter, you are initially shown the records of the patient in the lowest room number on the floor. To view the correct data for *your* patient, remember to select the correct room number, using the drop-down menu for the Patient field at the top left corner of the screen.

The EPR used in Pacific View Regional Hospital represents a composite of commercial versions being used in hospitals. You can access the EPR:

- to review existing data for a patient (by room number).
- to enter data you collect while working with a patient.

The EPR is updated daily, so no matter what day or part of a shift you are working, there will be a current EPR with the patient's data from the past days of the current hospital stay. This type of simulated EPR allows you to examine how data for different attributes have changed over time, as well as to examine data for all of a patient's attributes at a particular time. The EPR is fully functional (as it is in a real-life hospital). You can enter such data as blood pressure, breath sounds, and certain treatments. The EPR will not, however, allow you to enter data for a previous time period. Use the arrows at the bottom of the screen to move forward and backward in time.

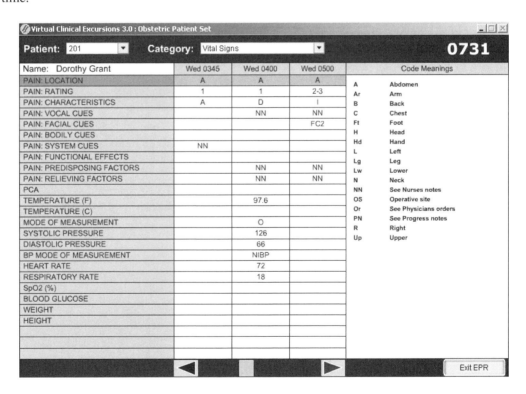

At the top of the EPR screen, you can choose patients by their room numbers. In addition, you have access to 17 different categories of patient data. To change patients or data categories, click the down arrow to the right of the room number or category.

The categories of patient data in the EPR are as follows:

- Vital Signs
- Respiratory
- Cardiovascular
- Neurologic
- Gastrointestinal
- Excretory
- Musculoskeletal
- Integumentary
- Reproductive
- Psychosocial
- Wounds and Drains
- Activity
- Hygiene and Comfort
- Safety
- Nutrition
- IV
- Intake and Output

Remember, each hospital selects its own codes. The codes used in the EPR at Pacific View Regional Hospital may be different from ones you have seen in your clinical rotations. Take some time to acquaint yourself with the codes. Within the Vital Signs category, click on any item in the left column (e.g., Pain: Characteristics). In the far-right column, you will see a list of code meanings for the possible findings and/or descriptors for that assessment area.

You will use the codes to record the data you collect as you work with patients. Click on the box in the last time column to the right of any item and wait for the code meanings applicable to that entry to appear. Select the appropriate code to describe your assessment findings and type it in the box. (*Note:* If no cursor appears within the box, click on the box again until the blue shading disappears and the blinking cursor appears.) Once the data are typed in this box, they are entered into the patient's record for this period of care only.

To leave the EPR, click on **Exit EPR** in the bottom right corner of the screen.

■ VISITING A PATIENT

From the Nurses' Station, click on the room number of the patient you wish to visit (in the tool bar at the bottom of your screen). Once you are inside the room, you will see a still photo of your patient in the top left corner. To verify that this is the correct patient, click on the **Check Armband** icon to the right of the photo. The patient's identification data will appear. If you click on **Check Allergies** (the next icon to the right), a list of the patient's allergies (if any) will replace the photo.

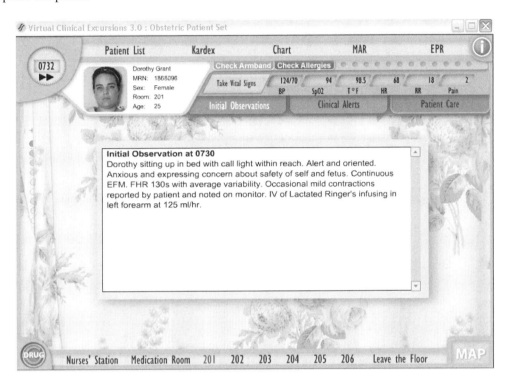

Also located in the patient's room are multiple icons you can use to assess the patient or the patient's medications. A virtual clock is provided in the upper left corner of the room to monitor your progress in real time. (*Note:* The fast-forward icon within the virtual clock will advance the time by 2-minute intervals when clicked.)

- The tool bar across the top of the screen allows you to check the **Patient List**, access the **EPR** to check or enter data, and view the patient's **Chart**, **MAR**, or **Kardex**.

- The **Take Vital Signs** icon allows you to measure the patient's up-to-the-minute blood pressure, oxygen saturation, temperature, heart rate, respiratory rate, and pain level.

- Each time you enter a patient's room, you are given an Initial Observation report to review (in the text box under the patient's photo). These notes are provided to give you a "look" at the patient as if you had just stepped into the room. You can also click on the **Initial Observations** icon to return to this box from other views within the patient's room. To the right of this icon is **Clinical Alerts**, a resource that allows you to make decisions about priority medication interventions based on emerging data collected in real time. Check this screen throughout your period of care to avoid missing critical information related to recently ordered or STAT medications.

- Clicking on **Patient Care** opens up three specific learning environments within the patient room: **Physical Assessment**, **Nurse-Client Interactions**, and **Medication Administration**.

- To perform a **Physical Assessment**, choose a body area (such as **Head & Neck**) from the column of yellow buttons. This activates a list of system subcategories for that body area (e.g., see **Sensory**, **Neurologic**, etc. in the green boxes). After you select the system you wish to evaluate, a brief description of the assessment findings will appear in a box to the right. A still photo provides a "snapshot" of how an assessment of this area might be done or what the finding might look like. For every body area, you can also click on **Equipment** on the right side of the screen.

- To the right of the Physical Assessment icon is **Nurse-Client Interactions**. Clicking on this icon will reveal the times and titles of any videos available for viewing. (*Note:* If the video you wish to see is not listed, this means you have not yet reached the correct virtual time to view that video. Check the virtual clock; you may return to access the video once its designated time has occurred—as long as you do so within the same period of care. Or you can click on the fast-forward icon within the virtual clock to advance the time by 2-minute intervals. You will then need to click again on **Patient Care** and **Nurse-Client Interactions** to refresh the screen.) To view a listed video, click on the white arrow to the right of the video title. Use the control buttons below the video to start, stop, pause, rewind, or fast-forward the action or to mute the sound.

- **Medication Administration** is the pathway that allows you to review and administer medications to a patient after you have prepared them in the Medication Room. This process is addressed further in *How to Prepare Medications* (pages 19-20), in *Medications* (pages 26-30), and in *Reducing Medication Errors* (pages 37-41).

■ HOW TO QUIT, CHANGE PATIENTS, OR CHANGE PERIODS OF CARE

How to Quit: From most screens, you may click the **Leave the Floor** icon on the bottom tool bar to the right of the patient room numbers. (*Note:* From some screens, you will first need to click an **Exit** button or **Return to Nurses' Station** before clicking **Leave the Floor**.) When the Floor Menu appears, click **Exit** to leave the program.

How to Change Patients or Periods of Care: To change patients, simply click on the new patient's room number. (You cannot receive a scorecard for a new patient, however, unless you have already selected that patient on the Patient List screen.) To change to a new period of care or to restart the virtual clock, click on **Leave the Floor** and then on **Restart the Program**.

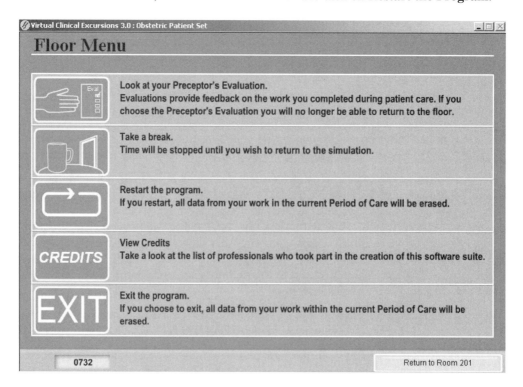

■ HOW TO PREPARE MEDICATIONS

From the Nurses' Station or the patient's room, you can access the Medication Room by clicking on the icon in the tool bar at the bottom of your screen to the left of the patient room numbers.

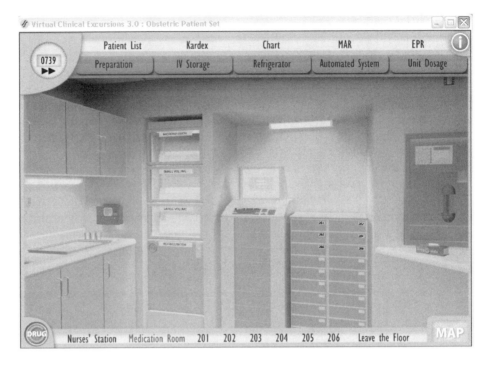

In the Medication Room you have access to the following (from left to right):

- A preparation area is located on the counter under the cabinets. To begin the medication preparation process, click on the tray on the counter or click on the **Preparation** icon at the top of the screen. The next screen leads you through a specific sequence (called the Preparation Wizard) to prepare medications one at a time for administration to a patient. However, no medication has been selected at this time. We will do this while working with a patient in *A Detailed Tour*. To exit this screen, click on **View Medication Room**.

- To the right of the cabinets (and above the refrigerator), IV storage bins are provided. Click on the bins themselves or on the **IV Storage** icon at the top of the screen. The bins are labeled **Microinfusion**, **Small Volume**, and **Large Volume**. Click on an individual bin to see a list of its contents. If you needed to prepare an IV medication at this time, you could click on the medication and its label would appear to the right under the patient's name. (*Note:* You can **Open** and **Close** any medication label by clicking the appropriate icon.) Next, you would click **Put Medication on Tray**. If you ever change your mind or decide that you have put the incorrect medication on the tray, you can reverse your actions by highlighting the medication on the tray and then clicking **Put Medication in Bin**. Click **Close Bin** in the right bottom corner to exit. **View Medication Room** brings you back to a full view of the entire room.

- A refrigerator is located under the IV storage bins to hold any medications that must be stored below room temperature. Click on the refrigerator door or on the **Refrigerator** icon at the top of the screen. Then click on the close-up view of the door to access the medications. When you are finished, click **Close Door** and then **View Medication Room**.

- To prepare controlled substances, click the **Automated System** icon at the top of the screen or click the computer monitor located to the right of the IV storage bins. A login screen will appear; your name and password are automatically filled in. Click **Login**. Select the patient for whom you wish to access medications; then select the correct medication drawer to open (they are stored alphabetically). Click **Open Drawer**, highlight the proper medication, and choose **Put Medication on Tray**. When you are finished, click **Close Drawer** and then **View Medication Room**.

- Next to the Automated System is a set of drawers identified by patient room number. To access these, click on the drawers or on the **Unit Dosage** icon at the top of the screen. This provides a close-up view of the drawers. To open a drawer, click on the room number of the patient you are working with. Next, click on the medication you would like to prepare for the patient, and a label will appear, listing the medication strength, units, and dosage per unit. To exit, click **Close Drawer**; then click **View Medication Room**.

At any time, you can learn about a medication you wish to prepare for a patient by clicking on the **Drug** icon in the bottom left corner of the medication room screen or by clicking the **Drug Guide** book on the counter to the right of the unit dosage drawers. The **Drug Guide** provides information about the medications commonly included in nursing drug handbooks. Nutritional supplements and maintenance intravenous fluid preparations are not included. Highlight a medication in the alphabetical list; relevant information about the drug will appear in the screen below. To exit, click **Return to Medication Room**.

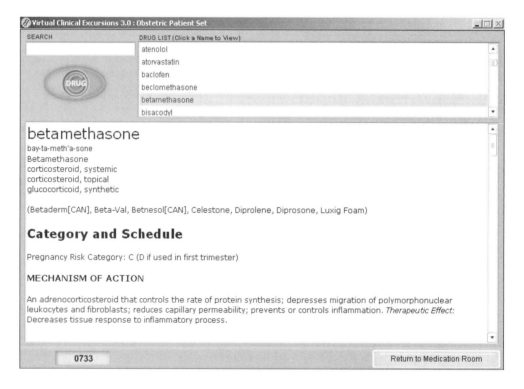

To access the MAR to review the medications ordered for a patient, click on the **MAR** icon located in the tool bar at the top of your screen and then click on the correct tab for your patient's room number. You may also click the **Review MAR** icon in the tool bar at the bottom of your screen from inside each medication storage area.

After you have chosen and prepared medications, go to the patient's room to administer them by clicking on the room number in the bottom tool bar. Inside the patient's room, click **Patient Care** and then **Medication Administration** and follow the proper administration sequence.

■ PRECEPTOR'S EVALUATIONS

When you have finished a session, click on **Leave the Floor** to go to the Floor Menu. At this point, you can click on the top icon (**Look at Your Preceptor's Evaluation**) to receive a scorecard that provides feedback on the work you completed during patient care.

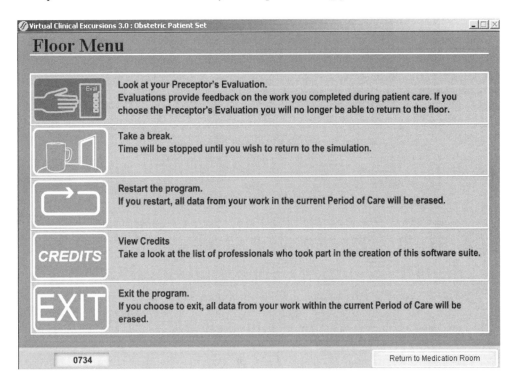

Evaluations are available for each patient you selected when you signed in for the current period of care. Click on the **Medication Scorecard** icon to see an example.

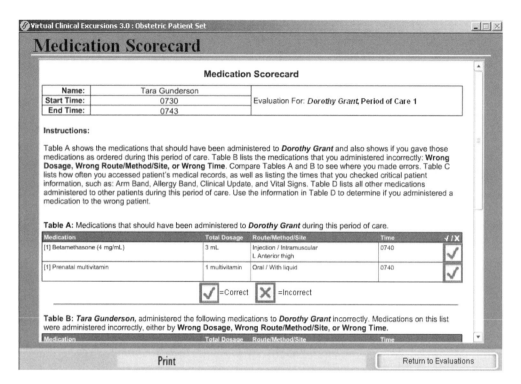

The scorecard compares the medications you administered to a patient during a period of care with what should have been administered. Table A lists the correct medications. Table B lists any medications that were administered incorrectly.

Remember, not every medication listed on the MAR should necessarily be given. For example, a patient might have an allergy to a drug that was ordered, or a medication might have been improperly transcribed to the MAR. Predetermined medication "errors" embedded within the program challenge you to exercise critical thinking skills and professional judgment when deciding to administer a medication, just as you would in a real hospital. Use all your available resources, such as the patient's chart and the MAR, to make your decision.

Table C lists the resources that were available to assist you in medication administration. It also documents whether and when you accessed these resources. For example, did you check the patient armband or perform a check of vital signs? If so, when?

You can click **Print** to get a copy of this report if needed. When you have finished reviewing the scorecard, click **Return to Evaluations** and then **Return to Menu**.

FLOOR MAP

To get a general sense of your location within the hospital, you can click on the **Map** icon found in the lower right corner of most of the screens in the *Virtual Clinical Excursions—Obstetrics* program. (*Note:* If you are following this quick tour step by step, you will need to **Restart the Program** from the Floor Menu, sign in again, and go to the Nurses' Station to access the map.) When you click the **Map** icon, a floor map appears, showing the layout of the floor you are currently on, as well as a directory of the patients and services on that floor. As you move your cursor over the directory list, the location of each room is highlighted on the map (and vice versa). The floor map can be accessed from the Nurses' Station, Medication Room, and each patient's room.

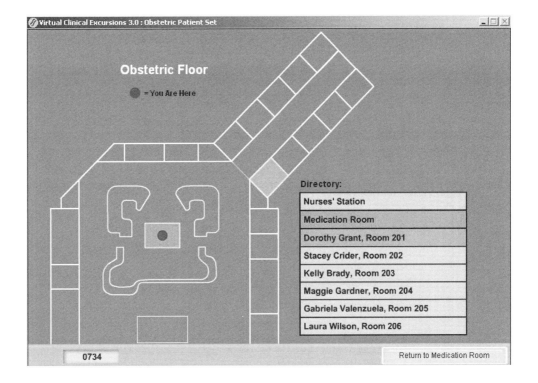

A DETAILED TOUR

If you wish to more thoroughly understand the capabilities of *Virtual Clinical Excursions—Obstetrics*, take a detailed tour by completing the following section. During this tour, we will work with a specific patient to introduce you to all the different components and learning opportunities available within the software.

■ WORKING WITH A PATIENT

Sign in for Period of Care 1 (0730-0815). From the Patient List, select Dorothy Grant in Room 201; however, do not go to the Nurses' Station yet.

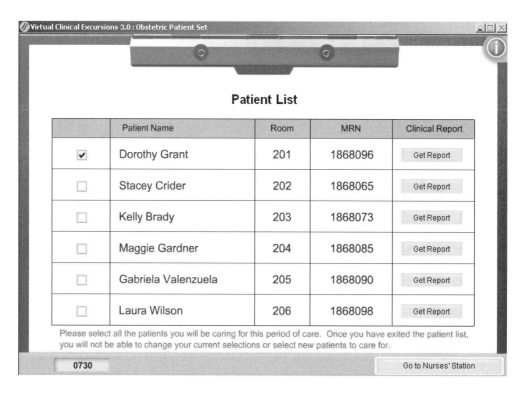

■ REPORT

In hospitals, when one shift ends and another begins, the outgoing nurse who attended a patient will give a verbal and sometimes a written summary of that patient's condition to the incoming nurse who will assume care for the patient. This summary is called a report and is an important source of data to provide an overview of a patient. Your first task is to get the clinical report on Dorothy Grant. To do this, click **Get Report** in the far right column in this patient's row. From a brief review of this summary, identify the problems and areas of concern that you will need to address for this patient.

When you have finished noting any areas of concern, click **Go to Nurses' Station**.

◼ CHARTS

You can access Dorothy Grant's chart from the Nurses' Station or from the patient's room (201). From the Nurses' Station, click on the chart rack or on the **Chart** icon in the tool bar at the top of your screen. Next, click on the chart labeled **201** to open the medical record for Dorothy Grant. Click on the **Emergency Department** tab to view a record of why this patient was admitted.

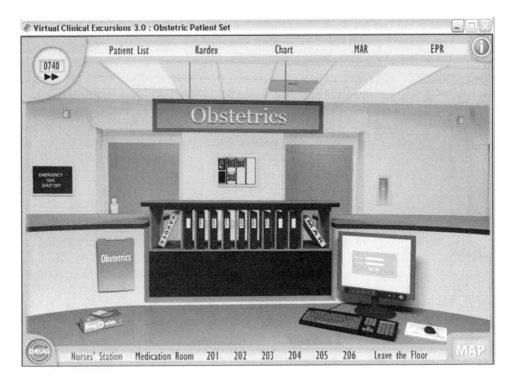

How many days has Dorothy Grant been in the hospital?

What tests were done upon her arrival in the Emergency Department and why?

What was the reason for her admission?

You should also click on **Surgical Reports** to learn whether any procedures were performed and when. Finally, review the **Nursing Admission** and **History and Physical** to learn about the health history of this patient. When you are done reviewing the chart, click **Return to Nurses' Station**.

■ MEDICATIONS

Open the Medication Administration Record (MAR) by clicking on the **MAR** icon in the tool bar at the top of your screen. *Remember:* The MAR automatically opens to the first occupied room number on the floor—which is not necessarily your patient's room number! Since you need to access Dorothy Grant's MAR, click on tab **201** (her room number). Always make sure you are giving the *Right Drug to the Right Patient!*

Examine the list of medications ordered for Dorothy Grant. In the table below, list the medications that need to be given during this period of care (0730-0815). For each medication, note the dosage, route, and time to be given.

Time	Medication	Dosage	Route

Click on **Return to Nurses' Station**. Next, click on **201** on the bottom tool bar and then verify that you are indeed in Dorothy Grant's room. Select **Clinical Alerts** (the icon to the right of Initial Observations) to check for any emerging data that might affect your medication administration priorities. Next, go to the patient's chart (click on the **Chart** icon; then click on **201**). When the chart opens, select the **Physician's Orders** tab.

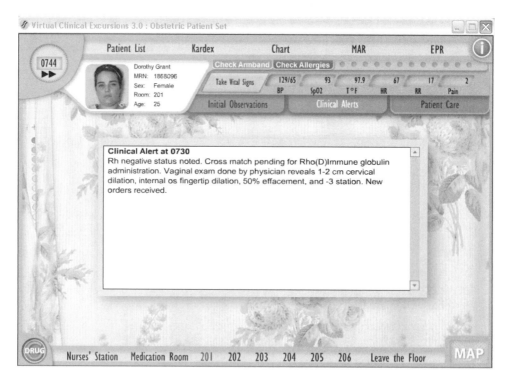

Review the orders. Have any new medications been ordered? Return to the MAR (click **Return to Room 201**; then click **MAR**). Verify that the new medications have been correctly transcribed to the MAR. Mistakes are sometimes made in the transcription process in the hospital setting, and it is sound practice to double-check any new order.

Are there any patient assessments you will need to perform before administering these medications? If so, return to Room 201 and click on **Patient Care** and then **Physical Assessment** to complete those assessments before proceeding.

Now click on the **Medication Room** icon in the tool bar at the bottom of your screen to locate and prepare the medications for Dorothy Grant.

In the Medication Room, you must access the medications for Dorothy Grant from the specific dispensing system in which each medication is stored. Locate each medication that needs to be given in this time period and click on **Put Medication on Tray** as appropriate. (*Hint:* Look in **Unit Dosage** drawer first.) When you are finished, click on **Close Drawer** and then on **View Medication Room**. Now click on the medication tray on the counter on the left side of the medication room screen to begin preparing the medications you have selected. (*Remember:* You can also click **Preparation** in the tool bar at the top of the screen.)

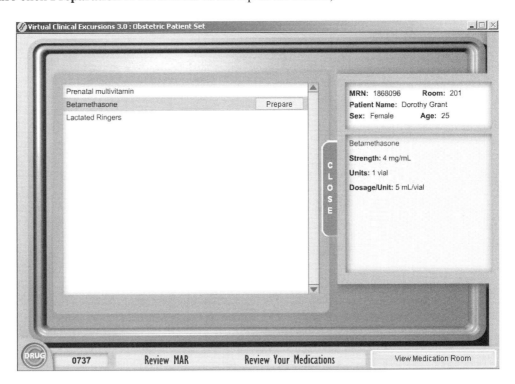

In the preparation area, you should see a list of the medications you put on the tray in the previous steps. Click on the first medication and then click **Prepare**. Follow the onscreen instructions of the Preparation Wizard, providing any data requested. As an example, let's follow the preparation process for betamethasone, one of the medications due to be administered to Dorothy Grant during this period of care. To begin, click on **Betamethasone**; then click **Prepare**. Now work through the Preparation Wizard sequence as detailed below:

> Amount of medication in the ampule: 5 mL.
> Enter the amount of medication you will draw up into a syringe: **3** mL.
> Click **Next**.
> Select the patient you wish to set aside the medication for: **Room 201, Dorothy Grant**.
> Click **Finish**.
> Click **Return to Medication Room**.

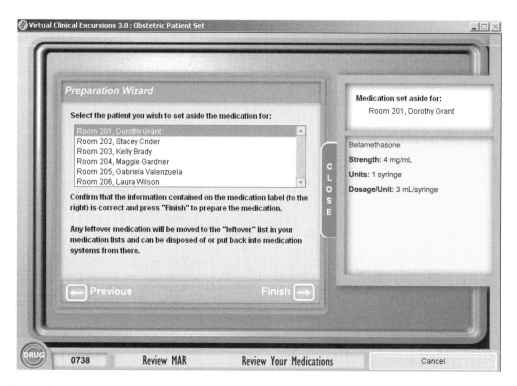

Follow this same basic process for the other medications due to be administered to Dorothy Grant during this period of care. (*Hint:* Look in **IV Storage** and **Automated System**.)

PREPARATION WIZARD EXCEPTIONS

- Some medications in *Virtual Clinical Excursions—Obstetrics* are prepared by the pharmacy (e.g., IV antibiotics) and taken to the patient room as a whole. This is common practice in most hospitals.
- Blood products are not administered by students through the *Virtual Clinical Excursions—Obstetrics* simulations since blood administration follows specific protocols not covered in this program.
- The *Virtual Clinical Excursions—Obstetrics* simulations do not allow for mixing more than one type of medication, such as regular and Lente insulins, in the same syringe. In the clinical setting, when multiple types of insulin are ordered for a patient, the regular insulin is drawn up first, followed by the longer-acting insulin. Insulin is always administered in a special unit-marked syringe.

Now return to Room 201 (click on **201** on the bottom tool bar) to administer Dorothy Grant's medications.

At any time during the medication administration process, you can perform a further review of systems, take vital signs, check information contained within the chart, or verify patient identity and allergies. Inside Dorothy Grant's room, click **Take Vital Signs**. (*Note:* These findings change over time to reflect the temporal changes you would find in a patient similar to Dorothy Grant.)

When you have gathered all the data you need, click on **Patient Care** and then select **Medication Administration**. Any medications you prepared in the previous steps should be listed on the left side of your screen. Let's continue the administration process with the betamethasone ordered for Dorothy Grant. Click to highlight **Betamethasone** in the list of medications. Next, click on the down arrow to the right of **Select** and choose **Administer** from the drop-down menu. This will activate the Administration Wizard. Complete the Wizard sequence as follows:

- Route: **Injection**
- Method: **Intramuscular**
- Site: **Any**
- Click **Administer to Patient** arrow.
- Would you like to document this administration in the MAR? **Yes**
- Click **Finish** arrow.

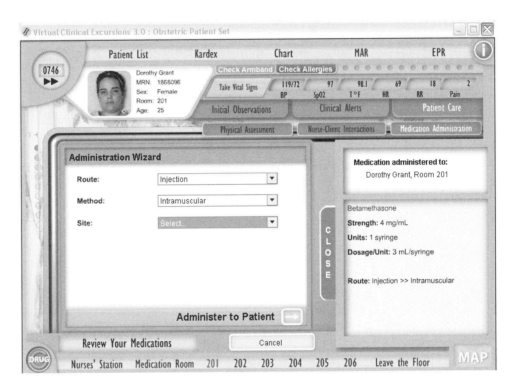

Your selections are recorded by a tracking system and evaluated on a Medication Scorecard stored under Preceptor's Evaluations. This scorecard can be viewed, printed, and given to your instructor. To access the Preceptor's Evaluations, click on **Leave the Floor**. When the Floor Menu appears, select **Look at Your Preceptor's Evaluation**. Then click on **Medication Scorecard** inside the box with Dorothy Grant's name (see example on the following page).

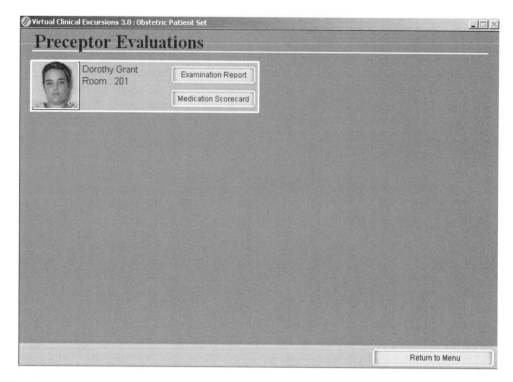

■ MEDICATION SCORECARD

- First, review Table A. Was betamethasone given correctly? Did you give the other medications as ordered?
- Table B shows you which (if any) medications you gave incorrectly.
- Table C addresses the resources used for Dorothy Grant. Did you access the patient's chart, MAR, EPR, or Kardex as needed to make safe medication administration decisions?
- Did you check the patient's armband to verify her identity? Did you check whether your patient had any known allergies to medications? Were vital signs taken?

When you have finished reviewing the scorecard, click **Return to Evaluations** and then **Return to Menu**.

■ VITAL SIGNS

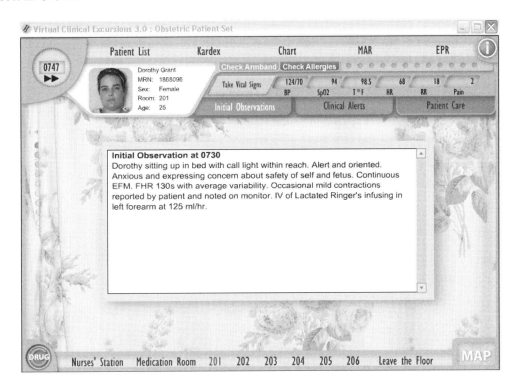

Vital signs, often considered the traditional "signs of life," include body temperature, heart rate, respiratory rate, blood pressure, oxygen saturation of the blood, and pain level.

Inside Dorothy Grant's room, click **Take Vital Signs**. (*Note:* If you are following this detailed tour step by step, you will need to **Restart the Program** from the Floor Menu, sign in again, and navigate to Room 201.) Collect vital signs for this patient and record them below. Note the time at which you collected each of these data. (*Remember:* You can take vital signs at any time. The data change over time to reflect the temporal changes you would find in a patient similar to Dorothy Grant.)

Vital Signs	Findings/Time
Blood pressure	
O$_2$ saturation	
Heart rate	
Respiratory rate	
Temperature	
Pain rating	

After you are done, click on the **EPR** icon located in the tool bar at the top of the screen. Your username and password are automatically provided. Click on **Login** to enter the EPR. To access Dorothy Grant's records, click on the down arrow next to Patient and choose her room number, **201**. Select **Vital Signs** as the category. Next, in the empty time column on the far right, record the vital signs data you just collected in the patient's room. (*Note:* If you need help with this process, see page 16.) Now compare these findings with the data you collected earlier for this patient's vital signs. Use these earlier findings to establish a baseline for each of the vital signs.

    a.   Are any of the data you collected significantly different from the baseline for a particular vital sign?

        Circle One: Yes   No

    b.   If "Yes," which data are different?

■ PHYSICAL ASSESSMENT

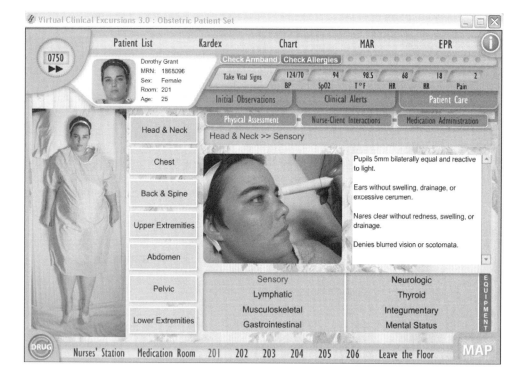

After you have finished examining the EPR for vital signs, click **Exit EPR** to return to Room 201. Click **Patient Care** and then **Physical Assessment**. Think about the information you received in the report at the beginning of this shift, as well as what you may have learned about this patient from the chart. Based on this, what area(s) of examination should you pay most attention to at this time? Is there any equipment you should be monitoring? Conduct a physical assessment of the body areas and systems that you consider priorities for Dorothy Grant. For example, select **Head & Neck**; then click on and assess **Sensory** and **Lymphatic**. Complete any other assessment(s) you think are necessary at this time. In the following table, record the data you collected during this examination.

Area of Examination	Findings
Head & Neck Sensory	
Head & Neck Lymphatic	

After you have finished collecting these data, return to the EPR. Compare the data that were already in the record with those you just collected.

   a.   Are any of the data you collected significantly different from the baselines for this patient?

        Circle One: Yes   No

   b.   If "Yes," which data are different?

■ **NURSE-CLIENT INTERACTIONS**

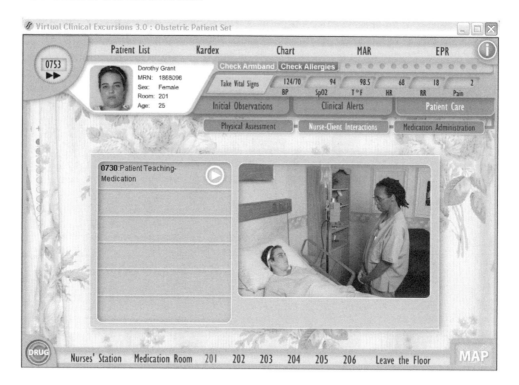

Click on **Patient Care** from inside Dorothy Grant's room (201). Now click on **Nurse-Client Interactions** to access a short video titled **Patient Teaching—Medication**, which is available for viewing at or after 0730 (based on the virtual clock in the upper left corner of your screen; see *Note* below). To begin the video, click on the white arrow next to its title. You will observe a nurse communicating with Dorothy Grant. There are many variations of nursing practice, some exemplifying "best" practice and some not. Note whether the nurse in this interaction displays professional behavior and compassionate care. Are her words congruent with what is going on with the patient? Does this interaction "feel right" to you? If not, how would you handle this situation differently? Explain.

Note: If the video you wish to view is not listed, this means you have not yet reached the correct virtual time to view that video. Check the virtual clock; you may return to access the video once its designated time has occurred—as long as you do so within the same period of care. Or you can click on the fast-forward icon within the virtual clock to advance the time by 2-minute intervals. You will then need to click again on **Patient Care** and **Nurse-Client Interactions** to refresh the screen.

At least one Nurse-Client Interactions video is available during each period of care. Viewing these videos can help you learn more about what is occurring with a patient at a certain time and also prompt you to discern between nurse communications that are ideal and those that need improvement. Compassionate care and the ability to communicate clearly are essential components of delivering quality nursing care, and it is during your clinical time that you will begin to refine these skills.

COLLECTING AND EVALUATING DATA

Each of the activities you perform in the Patient Care environment generates a significant amount of assessment data. Remember that after you collect data, you can record your findings in the EPR. You can also review the EPR, patient's chart, videos, and MAR at any time. You will get plenty of practice collecting and then evaluating data in context of the patient's course.

Now, here's an important question for you:

> Did the previous sequence of exercises provide the most efficient way to assess Dorothy Grant?

For example, you went to the patient's room to get vital signs, then back to the EPR to enter data and compare your findings with extant data. Next, you went back to the patient's room to do a physical examination, then again back to the EPR to enter and review data. If this back-and-forth process of data collection and recording seemed inefficient, remember the following:

- Plan all of your nursing activities to maximize efficiency, while at the same time optimizing the quality of patient care. (Think about what data you might need before performing certain tasks. For example, do you need to check a heart rate before administering a cardiac medication or check an IV site before starting an infusion?)

- You collect a tremendous amount of data when you work with a patient. Very few people can accurately remember all these data for more than a few minutes. Develop efficient assessment skills, and record data as soon as possible after collecting them.

- Assessment data are only the starting point for the nursing process.

Make a clear distinction between these first exercises and how you actually provide nursing care. These initial exercises were designed to involve you actively in the use of different software components. This workbook focuses on sensible practices for implementing the nursing process in ways that ensure the highest-quality care of patients.

Most important, remember that a human being changes through time, and that these changes include both the physical and psychosocial facets of a person as a living organism. Think about this for a moment. Some patients may change physically in a very short time (a patient with emerging myocardial infarction) or more slowly (a patient with a chronic illness). Patients' overall physical and psychosocial conditions may improve or deteriorate. They may have effective coping skills and familial support, or they may feel alone and full of despair. In fact, each individual is a complex mix of physical and psychosocial elements, and at least some of these elements usually change through time.

Thus it is crucial that you *DO NOT* think of the nursing process as a simple one-time, five-step procedure consisting of assessment, nursing diagnosis, planning, implementation, and evaluation. Rather, the nursing process should be utilized as a creative and systematic approach to delivering nursing care. Furthermore, because all living organisms are constantly changing, we must apply the nursing process over and over. Each time we follow the nursing process for an individual patient, we refine our understanding of that patient's physical and psychosocial conditions based on collection and analysis of many different types of data. *Virtual Clinical Excursions—Obstetrics* will help you develop both the creativity and the systematic approach needed to become a nurse who is equipped to deliver the highest-quality care to all patients.

REDUCING MEDICATION ERRORS

Earlier in this detailed tour, you learned the basic steps of medication preparation and administration. The following simulations will allow you to practice those skills further—with an increased emphasis on reducing medication errors by using the Medication Scorecard to evaluate your work.

Sign in to work at Pacific View Regional Hospital for Period of Care 1. (*Note:* If you are already working with another patient or during another period of care, click on **Leave the Floor** and then **Restart the Program**; then sign in.)

From the Patient List, select Dorothy Grant. Then click on **Go to Nurses' Station**. Complete the following steps to prepare and administer medications to Dorothy Grant.

- Click on **Medication Room**.
- Click on **MAR** and then on tab **201** to determine prn medications that have been ordered for Dorothy Grant. (*Note:* You may click on **Review MAR** at any time to verify the correct medication order. Always remember to check the patient name on the MAR to make sure you have the correct patient's record—you must click on the correct room number tab within the MAR.) Click on **Return to Medication Room** after reviewing the correct MAR.
- Click on **Unit Dosage** (or on the Unit Dosage cabinet); from the close-up view, click on drawer **201**.
- Select the medications you would like to administer. After each selection, click **Put Medication on Tray**. When you are finished selecting medications, click **Close Drawer** and then **View Medication Room**.
- Click **Automated System** (or on the Automated System unit itself). Click **Login**.
- On the next screen, specify the correct patient and drawer location.
- Select the medication you would like to administer and click **Put Medication on Tray**. Repeat this process if you wish to administer other medications from the Automated System.
- When you are finished, click **Close Drawer** and **View Medication Room**.
- From the Medication Room, click **Preparation** (or on the preparation tray).
- From the list of medications on your tray, highlight the correct medication to administer and click **Prepare**.
- This activates the Preparation Wizard. Supply any requested information; then click **Next**.
- Now select the correct patient to receive this medication and click **Finish**.
- Repeat the previous three steps until all medications that you want to administer are prepared.
- You can click on **Review Your Medications** and then on **Return to Medication Room** when ready. Once you are back in the Medication Room, go directly to Dorothy Grant's room by clicking on **201** at the bottom of the screen.
- Inside the patient's room, administer the medication, utilizing the five rights of medication administration. After you have collected the appropriate assessment data and are ready for administration, click **Patient Care** and then **Medication Administration**. Verify that the correct patient and medication(s) appear in the left-hand window. Highlight the first medication you wish to administer; then click the down arrow next to Select. From the drop-down menu, select **Administer** and complete the Administration Wizard by providing any information requested. When the Wizard stops asking for information, click **Administer to Patient**. Specify **Yes** when asked whether this administration should be recorded in the MAR. Finally, click **Finish**.

■ SELF-EVALUATION

Now let's see how you did during your medication administration!

- Click on **Leave the Floor** at the bottom of your screen. From the Floor Menu, select **Look at Your Preceptor's Evaluation**. Then click **Medication Scorecard**.

The following exercises will help you identify medication errors, investigate possible reasons for these errors, and reduce or prevent medication errors in the future.

1. Start by examining Table A. These are the medications you should have given to Dorothy Grant during this period of care. If each of the medications in Table A has a ✓ by it, then you made no errors. Congratulations!

If any medication has an X by it, then you made one or more medication errors.

Compare Tables A and B to determine which of the following types of errors you made: Wrong Dose, Wrong Route/Method/Site, or Wrong Time. Follow these steps:
   a. Find medications in Table A that were given incorrectly.
   b. Now see if those same medications are in Table B, which shows what you actually administered to Dorothy Grant.
   c. Comparing Tables A and B, match the Strength, Dose, Route/Method/Site, and Time for each medication you administered incorrectly.
   d. Then, using the form below, list the medications given incorrectly and mark the errors you made for each medication.

Medication	Strength	Dosage	Route	Method	Site	Time
	❑	❑	❑	❑	❑	❑
	❑	❑	❑	❑	❑	❑
	❑	❑	❑	❑	❑	❑
	❑	❑	❑	❑	❑	❑

2. To help you reduce future medication errors, consider the following list of possible reasons for errors.

- Did not check drug against MAR for correct patient, correct date, correct time, correct drug, and correct dose.
- Did not check drug dose against MAR three times.
- Did not open the unit dose package in the patient's room.
- Did not correctly identify the patient using two identifiers.
- Did not administer the drug on time.
- Did not verify patient allergies.
- Did not check the patient's current condition or vital sign parameters.
- Did not consider why the patient would be receiving this drug.
- Did not question why the drug was in the patient's drawer.
- Did not check the physician's order and/or check with the pharmacist when there was a question about the drug or dose.
- Did not verify that no adverse effects had occurred from a previous dose.

Based on the list of possibilities you just reviewed, determine how you made each error and record the reason in the form below:

Medication	Reason for Error

3. Look again at Table B. Are there medications listed that are not in Table A? If so, you gave a medication to Dorothy Grant that she should not have received. Complete the following exercises to help you understand how such an error might have been made.

   a. Perhaps you gave a medication that was on Dorothy Grant's MAR for this period of care, without recognizing that a change had occurred in the patient's condition, which should have caused you to reconsider. Review patient records as necessary and complete the following form:

Medication	Possible Reasons Not to Give This Medication

   b. Another possibility is that you gave Dorothy Grant a medication that should have been given at a different time. Check her MAR and complete the form below to determine whether you made a Wrong Time error:

Medication	Given to Dorothy Grant at What Time	Should Have Been Given at What Time

c. Maybe you gave another patient's medication to Dorothy Grant. In this case, you made a Wrong Patient error. Check the MARs of other patients and use the form below to determine whether you made this type of error:

Medication	Given to Dorothy Grant	Should Have Been Given to

4. The Medication Scorecard provides some other interesting sources of information. For example, if there is a medication selected for Dorothy Grant but it was not given to her, there will be an X by that medication in Table A, but it will not appear in Table B. In that case, you might have given this medication to some other patient, which is another type of Wrong Patient error. To investigate further, look at Table D, which lists the medications you gave to other patients. See whether you can find any medications ordered for Dorothy Grant that were given to another patient by mistake. However, before you make any decisions, be sure to cross-check the MAR for other patients because the same medication may have been ordered for multiple patients. Use the following form to record your findings:

Medication	Should Have Been Given to Dorothy Grant	Given by Mistake to

5. Now take some time to review the medication exercises you just completed. Use the form below to create an overall analysis of what you have learned. Once again, record each of the medication errors you made, including the type of each error. Then, for each error you made, indicate specifically what you would do differently to prevent this type of error from occurring again.

Medication	Type of Error	Error Prevention Tactic

Submit this form to your instructor if required as a graded assignment, or simply use these exercises to improve your understanding of medication errors and how to reduce them.

Name: _____   Date: _____

The following icons are used throughout this workbook to help you quickly identify particular activities and assignments:

 Indicates a reading assignment—tells you which textbook chapter(s) you should read before starting each lesson

 Indicates a writing activity

 Marks the beginning of an interactive CD-ROM activity—signals you to open or return to your *Virtual Clinical Excursions—Obstetrics* CD-ROM

 Indicates additional CD-ROM instructions

 Indicates questions and activities that require you to consult your textbook

 Indicates the approximate time required to complete an exercise

LESSON **1**

Assessment and Health Promotion

Reading Assignment: Assessment and Health Promotion (Chapter 2)

Patients: Maggie Gardner, Room 204
Gabriela Valenzuela, Room 205
Laura Wilson, Room 206

Goal: Identify the variations found in the pregnant patient's assessment, including health risk behaviors and health promotion techniques to assist in the optimal outcome for the fetus.

Objectives:

- Discuss the variations in a pregnant patient's assessment findings.
- Identify health risks in pregnant patients.
- Explore health promotion interventions that can and/or should be completed by the nurse caring for those patients with high-risk behaviors.

Exercise 1

 CD-ROM Activity

 30 minutes

- Sign in to work at Pacific View Regional Hospital on the Obstetrics Floor for Period of Care 1. (*Note:* If you are already in the virtual hospital from a previous exercise, click on **Leave the Floor** and then on **Restart the Program** to get to the sign-in window.)
- From the Patient List, select Maggie Gardner (Room 204).
- Click on **Go to Nurses' Station**.
- Click on **204** at the bottom of the screen.
- Inside the patient's room, click on **Patient Care**.
- Click on the **Physical Assessment** tab.
- Click on the **Chest** section.
- Click on the box labeled **Breasts** and note the assessment findings.

1. According to the textbook, what are the normal findings on a breast assessment?

2. Compare the normal assessment findings listed in the textbook with Maggie Gardner's breast assessment findings.

→ • From Maggie Gardner's room, click on **Chart** at the top of the screen.
 • Click on **204** to open her chart.
 • Click on **Nursing Admission**.
 • Review question 13 on page 5 of the **Nursing Admission**.

As a part of your health promotion for this patient, answer the following questions.

3. Does Maggie Gardner do monthly breast self-exams?

4. Has she ever had a mammogram?

5. According to the textbook, what is the recommendation regarding mammograms and Maggie Gardner's age group?

6. According to the textbook, what should Maggie Gardner be taught about breast self-examination?

According to the textbook, there are many barriers to seeking health care. As you can see, this is true for Maggie Gardner. Answer the following questions regarding these barriers. (*Hint:* If you have closed the chart, reopen it and return to the Nursing Admission section.)

 7. List three barriers to seeking health care, as identified in Chapter 2 of the textbook.

8. Maggie Gardner identifies the barrier that prevented her from seeking health care and keeping her appointments. What was that barrier? (*Hint:* See the Nursing Admission form in the chart.)

Exercise 2

 CD-ROM Activity

 45 minutes

Barriers to getting health care can be coupled with risks during the childbearing years. In this section, we will focus on another patient, Laura Wilson.

- Sign in to work at Pacific View Regional Hospital on the Obstetrics Floor for Period of Care 3. (*Note:* If you are already in the virtual hospital from a previous exercise, click on **Leave the Floor** and then on **Restart the Program** to get to the sign-in window.)
- From the Patient List, select Laura Wilson (Room 206).
- Click on **Go to Nurses' Station**.
- Click on **Chart** and then on **206**.
- Click on the **History and Physical** or the **Nursing Admission** tab to answer the following questions.

1. List the factors that put Laura Wilson at risk during her pregnancy.

2. From the Nursing Admission, what does Laura Wilson say about her drug use, smoking, and alcohol use in regard to her pregnancy and the outcome for her baby?

- Click on **Return to Nurses' Station**.
- Click on **206** at the bottom of the screen.
- Click on **Patient Care** and then on **Nurse-Client Interactions**.
- Select and view the video titled **1530: Discharge Planning**. Make some notes about this interaction to use for answering questions later. (*Note:* Check the virtual clock to see whether enough time has elapsed. You can use the fast-forward feature to advance the time by 2-minute intervals if the video is not yet available. Then click again on **Patient Care** and **Nurse-Client Interactions** to refresh the screen.)
- Now click on **Nurses' Station** at the bottom of the screen.
- Click on **Chart** and then on **206**.
- Click on the **Consultations** tab and review the Psychiatric Consult. (*Note:* If this document does not appear when you open the Consultations tab, check the virtual clock to see whether enough time has elapsed. This Psychiatric Consult is not available until 1530. You can use the fast-forward feature to advance the time by 2-minute intervals if the note is not yet available. You may need to close and reopen the chart to "refresh" the contents.)

Answer the following questions based on your impression of the 1530 video interaction and the observations made in the Psychiatric Consult.

3. In the Psychiatric Consult, what was the clinician's perspective of Laura Wilson in relation to her current life situation?

4. Based on the video interaction, what is your impression of Laura Wilson?

5. What does Laura Wilson say that indicates she may not understand HIV or is in denial that it is truly a medical concern? (*Hint:* Read the Nurse's Notes in her chart.)

6. Based on your review of the 1530 video interaction and the Psychiatric Consult, what areas of health education (health promotion) need to be the focus for Laura Wilson?

Exercise 3

 CD-ROM Activity

 30 minutes

The head-to-toe assessment is a key part of obtaining data, both subjective and objective, from our patients. The following exercise will walk you through an assessment on an obstetric patient. The goal of this exercise is to identify abnormal findings or pregnancy-related changes in each of the body systems.

- Sign in to work at Pacific View Regional Hospital on the Obstetrics Floor for Period of Care 2. (*Note:* If you are already in the virtual hospital from a previous exercise, click on **Leave the Floor** and then on **Restart the Program** to get to the sign-in window.)
- From the Patient List, select Gabriela Valenzuela (Room 205).
- Click on **Go to Nurses' Station**.
- Click on **205** at the bottom of the screen.
- Click on **Patient Care** and then on **Physical Assessment**.
- One at a time, click on the various body areas (yellow buttons) and the subsystems (green boxes) to complete the head-to-toe assessment.

1. Under each of the body areas below, list any abnormal findings or changes related to pregnancy gathered from your physical assessment of Gabriela Valenzuela.

Head & Neck

Chest

Back & Spine

Upper Extremities

Abdomen

Pelvic

Lower Extremities

2. Once the health assessment is complete, what is the nurse's responsibility to these patients on their return visits?

3. List five areas in which a nurse needs to educate women to help them maintain healthy lives.

4. Pelvic exams are recommended _____ until women are _____ years

   old. These exams are to be started whenever a female _____.

5. Holli, a 65-year-old, states that she hates going to the doctor because they always seem to be males. However, she needs to have a physical exam because it has been "years" since her last one. Based on your reading, how could you help this woman overcome the barriers that she has to health care? Also, what information could you provide to her that would help her be prepared for the examination?

LESSON 2

Substance Abuse/ Violence Against Women

___

 Reading Assignment: Assessment and Health Promotion (Chapter 2)

Patients: Dorothy Grant, Room 201
Laura Wilson, Room 206

Goals: Identify patients at risk for intimate partner violence, interventions to assist those at risk, and ways to educate and empower those individuals toward healthy relationships; demonstrate an understanding of the identification of substance abuse issues in pregnant women.

Objectives:

- Assess and plan care for a substance-abusing woman with a term pregnancy.
- Discuss the statistics related to intimate partner violence (IPV).
- List characteristics of battered women.
- Explore the myths and facts regarding IPV.
- Identify the nurse's role in regard to battered women or those involved in IPV.

Exercise 1

 CD-ROM Activity

🕐 30 minutes

- Sign in to work at Pacific View Regional Hospital on the Obstetrics Floor for Period of Care 2. (*Note*: If you are already in the virtual hospital from a previous exercise, click on **Leave the Floor** and then on **Restart the Program** to get to the sign-in window.)
- From the Patient List, select Laura Wilson (Room 206).
- Click on **Go to Nurses' Station**.
- Click on **Chart** and then on **206**.
- Click on **Nursing Admission**.

1. Complete the table below with information on Laura Wilson's use of tobacco, alcohol, and illicit drugs. (*Hint:* Refer to page 4 of the Nursing Admission.)

Substance	Reported Use
Tobacco	
Alcohol	
Marijuana	
Crack cocaine	

 Read about tobacco, alcohol, marijuana, and cocaine in the section on Substance Abuse and Use on pages 39-40 in your textbook.

2. Complete the table below by placing an X beneath the substance(s) thought to be associated with each of the listed pregnancy-related risks.

Pregnancy-Related Risk	Tobacco	Alcohol	Marijuana	Cocaine
Miscarriage				
Placental perfusion abnormalities				
Premature rupture of membranes				
Preterm labor/birth				
Placenta previa				
Abruptio placentae				
Chorioamnionitis				
Fetal alcohol syndrome (FAS)				
Fetal alcohol effects (FAE)				
Hypertension				
Stillbirth				
Anemia				
Fetal abnormalities				
Low birth weight or fetal growth restriction				
Mental retardation/ developmental problems (child)				

• Click on **Return to Nurses' Station**.
 • Click on **206** at the bottom of the screen.
 • Click on **Patient Care** and then on **Nurse-Client Interactions**.
 • Select and view the video titled **1115: Teaching—Effects of Drug Use**. (*Note:* Check the virtual clock to see whether enough time has elapsed. You can use the fast-forward feature to advance the time by 2-minute intervals if the video is not yet available. Then click again on **Patient Care** and **Nurse-Client Interactions** to refresh the screen.)

3. Does Laura Wilson consider herself to be addicted? Support your answer with comments from the video interactions.

4. How does Laura Wilson think her drug use will affect the baby?

5. According to the nurse in the video interaction, how might Laura Wilson's drug use affect the baby?

6. Review the following list of nursing interventions to deal with Laura Wilson's drug use. Place an X next to the intervention(s) you believe would be most appropriate at this time. Select all that apply.

   _____ Talk with Laura Wilson in a manner that conveys caring and concern.

   _____ Urge Laura Wilson to begin a drug treatment program today.

   _____ Explain to Laura Wilson that she may lose custody of her baby if her drug use continues.

   _____ Involve other members of the health care team in Laura Wilson's care.

7. Explain the choice(s) you made in question 6.

Exercise 2

 CD-ROM Activity

 45 minutes

 Before beginning this CD-ROM activity, answer the following questions based on your review of pages 42-44 in your textbook.

    1. _____ million women each year are affected by violence against women.

    2. IPV is the _____ leading cause of injuries in women age _____ in the United States.

• Sign in to work at Pacific View Regional Hospital on the Obstetrics Floor for Period of Care 1. (*Note*: If you are already in the virtual hospital from a previous exercise, click on **Leave the Floor** and then on **Restart the Program** to get to the sign-in window.)
• From the Patient List, select Dorothy Grant (Room 201).
• Click on **Go to Nurses' Station**.
• Click on **Chart** and then on **201**.
• Click on the **Nursing Admission** tab.

 Review the Nursing Admission for Dorothy Grant's perspective of the abusive relationship that she has experienced. Then review the characteristics of battered women described on page 44 in your textbook. Answer the following questions.

    3. What is the reality of Dorothy Grant's situation (based on the Nursing Admission)? How does that correlate with what you learned in the textbook reading?

 • Click on **Return to Room 201**.
• Click on **201** at the bottom of the screen.
• Click on **Patient Care** and then on **Nurse-Client Interactions**.
• Select and view the video titled **0810: Monitoring/Patient Support**. (*Note:* Check the virtual clock to see whether enough time has elapsed. You can use the fast-forward feature to advance the time by 2-minute intervals if the video is not yet available. Then click again on **Patient Care** and **Nurse-Client Interactions** to refresh the screen.)

4. In the video interaction, what does Dorothy Grant say that she should do to help keep the violence away?

5. In the video interaction, what are the patient's concerns at the moment?

➡ • Click on **Chart** and then on **201**.
   • Click on the **History and Physical** tab and review.
   • Click on the **Nursing Admission** and review.

6. According to the textbook, battered women have certain characteristics (listed in the table below and on the next page). Compare this list with what you have learned about Dorothy Grant in her chart and through the 0810 nurse-client interaction you observed earlier. Mark an X next to each characteristic that applies to Dorothy Grant. When appropriate, support your choice with documentation from the chart or video.

Financially dependent

Blames self for what has taken place

States that she is "not good enough"

Low self-esteem

History of domestic violence in her family

Fears societal rejection

Attempts to avoid arousing anger in the abuser

Deliberate/repeated physical or sexual assault

Now let's jump ahead in virtual time to review Dorothy Grant's records from a later period of care.

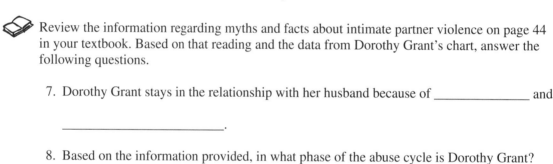

• Sign in to work at Pacific View Regional Hospital on the Obstetrics Floor for Period of Care 3. (*Note*: If you are already in the virtual hospital from a previous exercise, click on **Leave the Floor** and then **Restart the Program** to get to the sign-in window.)
• From the Patient List, select Dorothy Grant (Room 201).
• Click on **Go to Nurses' Station**.
• Click on **Chart** and then on **201**.
• Click on **Consultations** and review the Psychiatric Consult and the Social Work Consult.

Review the information regarding myths and facts about intimate partner violence on page 44 in your textbook. Based on that reading and the data from Dorothy Grant's chart, answer the following questions.

7. Dorothy Grant stays in the relationship with her husband because of _____ and

    _____.

8. Based on the information provided, in what phase of the abuse cycle is Dorothy Grant?

9. According to the consultation reports, Dorothy Grant has several options. What are some of the options that the social worker and psychiatric heath care provider can offer her or assist her with?

10. Indicate whether each of the following statements is true or false.

    a. _____ Battering often escalates or begins during pregnancy.

    b. _____ Dorothy Grant's husband blames her for the pregnancy.

    c. _____ Dorothy Grant stays in the abusive relationship because she likes to be beaten and deliberately provokes the attacks on occasion.

Exercise 3

 CD-ROM Activity

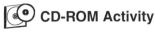 20 minutes

- Sign in to work at Pacific View Regional Hospital on the Obstetrics Floor for Period of Care 4. (*Note*: If you are already in the virtual hospital from a previous exercise, click on **Leave the Floor** and then on **Restart the Program** to get to the sign-in window.)
- Click on **Kardex** at the top of the screen and then tab **201** to review Dorothy Grant's record. (*Remember:* You are not able to visit patients or administer medications during Period of Care 4. You are only able to review patients' records.)

1. What action was initiated on Wednesday to protect Dorothy Grant from her husband?

2. What care plan diagnoses are appropriate for Dorothy Grant's current life situation?

3. Members of what other disciplines have been contacted or consulted to ensure continuity of care for Dorothy Grant as it relates to her abuse?

4. As a nurse caring for Dorothy Grant, what is your responsibility for reporting IPV?

5. What are the reporting requirements of the state in which you practice?

6. What are the resources available in your area for women who are experiencing intimate partner violence?

Sexually Transmitted and Other Infections

 Reading Assignment: Common Concerns (Chapter 3)

Pregnancy at Risk: Gestational Considerations (Chapter 21)

Patients: Stacey Crider, Room 202

Gabriela Valenzuela, Room 205

Laura Wilson, Room 206

Goal: Demonstrate an understanding of the identification and management of selected sexually transmitted and other infections in pregnant women.

Objectives:

• Assess and plan care for a pregnant woman with bacterial vaginosis.

• Explain the importance of prophylactic Group B streptococcus treatment.

• Identify risk factors for acquiring HIV infection.

• Prioritize information to be included in patient teaching related to HIV infection.

In this lesson you will assess and evaluate the care provided to three hospitalized pregnant women, each of whom has or is at risk for having a sexually transmitted infection (STI).

Exercise 1

 Writing Activity

5 minutes

1. A patient reports to the physician with complaints consistent with chlamydia. Upon confirmation of the infection, which of the following medications will most likely be prescribed?
   a. Azithromycin orally for 7 days
   b. Doxycycline orally for 7 days
   c. Metronidazole vaginal suppositories for 3 days
   d. Ceftriaxone one dose IM

2. A pregnant woman fears that she has been exposed to syphilis. Which of the following manifestations is consistent with this disease?
   a. A painless ulceration
   b. A painful, weeping vesicle
   c. A diffuse red rash
   d. Several flesh-colored growths on the perineum

3. The most common group to become infected with genital herpes simplex is women ages

   _____ to _____ years.

4. Indicate whether each of the following statements is true or false.

   a. _____ The use of corticosteroids is associated with an increased incidence of candidiasis infection.

   b. _____ Trichomoniasis is often diagnosed with the Pap test.

Exercise 2

CD-ROM Activity

15 minutes

- Sign in to work at Pacific View Regional Hospital on the Obstetrics Floor for Period of Care 1. (*Note*: If you are already in the virtual hospital from a previous exercise, click on **Leave the Floor** and then on **Restart the Program** to get to the sign-in window.)
- From the Patient List, select Stacey Crider (Room 202).
- Click on **Go to Nurses' Station**.
- Click on **Chart** and then on **202**.
- Click on **History and Physical**.

Read about bacterial vaginosis on page 82 (Table 3-3) in your textbook.

1. In the table below, describe Stacey Crider's vaginal discharge on admission. How does it compare with the description of bacterial vaginosis found in your textbook?

	Stacey Crider's Discharge	Textbook Description
Appearance		
Amount		
Odor		

2. When the patient presents with symptoms consistent with bacterial vaginosis, what diagnostic test result will confirm the presence of the infection?
   a. Presence of many white blood cell protozoa with a saline wet smear
   b. Presence of hyphae and pseudohyphae with a saline wet smear
   c. Presence of clue cells with a saline wet smear
   d. Release of a fishy odor when mixed with normal saline

3. A patient who is 12 weeks pregnant has been diagnosed with bacterial vaginosis. What is the recommended treatment?
   a. Metronidazole (Flagyl)
   b. Tetracycline
   c. Gyne-Lotrimin
   d. Amoxicillin

→ • Now click on **Physician's Orders**.
  • Scroll down to the admitting physician's orders on Tuesday at 0630.

4. What are Stacey Crider's admission diagnoses?

5. Explain how Stacey Crider's admission diagnoses are likely to be related.

6. Which medication did Stacey Crider's physician order to treat her bacterial vaginosis?

7. When providing teaching to Stacey Crider concerning the medication prescribed to treat her bacterial vaginosis, what potential side effects should be included in the education provided? Select all that apply.

   _____ Nausea

   _____ Vomiting

   _____ Diarrhea

   _____ Furry tongue

   _____ Fatigue

8. Indicate whether each of the following statements is true or false.

a. _____ Stacey Crider's sexual partners should be treated for the infection.

b. _____ Stacey Crider's physician will be required to report a listing of her sexual partners to the Department of Health as a result of her vaginal infection.

Exercise 3

CD-ROM Activity

30 minutes

- Sign in to work at Pacific View Regional Hospital on the Obstetrics Floor for Period of Care 1. (*Note*: If you are already in the virtual hospital from a previous exercise, click on **Leave the Floor** and then on **Restart the Program** to get to the sign-in window.)
- From the Patient List, select Gabriela Valenzuela (Room 205).
- Click on **Go to Nurses' Station**.
- Click on **Chart** and then on **205**.
- Click on **History and Physical** and scroll to the plan at the end of this document.

1. What is the medical plan of care for Gabriela Valenzuela?

2. Is Gabriela Valenzuela known to be positive for Group B streptococcus (GBS)?

3. List risk factors for neonatal GBS infection. Place an X by each factor that applies to Gabriela Valenzuela.

4. Since pregnant women with GBS in the vagina are almost always asymptomatic, why does Gabriela Valenzuela need to be treated for this organism?

5. _____ Nonpregnant women who are diagnosed with GBS must be treated to avoid further complications. (True/False)

→ • Click on **Physician's Orders**.
  • Scroll to the admission orders written Tuesday at 2100.

6. What medication/dosage/frequency will Gabriela Valenzuela receive for Group B strep prophylaxis?

Consult Table 21-9 on pages 661-662 in your textbook; then answer question 7.

7. How does the physician's order you identified in question 6 compare with the treatment regimen recommended in your textbook?

Exercise 4

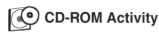 **CD-ROM Activity**

 30 minutes

- Sign in to work at Pacific View Regional Hospital on the Obstetrics Floor for Period of Care 1. (*Note*: If you are already in the virtual hospital from a previous exercise, click on **Leave the Floor** and then on **Restart the Program** to get to the sign-in window.)
- From the Patient List, select Laura Wilson (Room 206).
- Click on **Go to Nurses' Station**.
- Click on **Chart** and then on **206**.
- Click on **Nursing Admission**.

1. What risk factors for acquiring an STI are identified on Laura Wilson's Nursing Admission form?

 Read about human immunodeficiency virus (HIV) on pages 79-82 in your textbook.

2. List specific risk factors for acquiring HIV infection. Place an X by each risk factor that applies to Laura Wilson's history.

3. What did the admitting nurse document about Laura Wilson's knowledge and acceptance of her HIV diagnosis?

• Click on **Return to Nurses' Station** and then on **206** at the bottom of the screen.
   • Click on **Patient Care** and then on **Nurse-Client Interactions**.
   • Select and view the video titled **0800: Teaching—HIV in Pregnancy**. (*Note:* Check the virtual clock to see whether enough time has elapsed. You can use the fast-forward feature to advance the time by 2-minute intervals if the video is not yet available. Then click again on **Patient Care** and **Nurse-Client Interactions** to refresh the screen.)

4. Does Laura Wilson appear to be fully aware of the implications of HIV infection? State the rationale for your answer.

5. What coping mechanism is Laura Wilson exhibiting in the video interaction?

 • Click on **Chart** and then on **206**.
   • Click on **Nursing Admission**.

6. Laura Wilson needs education on all of the following topics. Which would you choose to teach her about at this particular time?
   a. Safer sex
   b. Medication side effects and importance of compliance
   c. Need for medical follow-up and medication for the baby
   d. Impact of HIV on birth plans

7. Give a rationale for your answer to question 6.

8. Which of the following statistics best represents the risk for transmission of HIV to a baby born to an HIV-positive mother when treatment is implemented during the pregnancy?
   a. Less than 3%
   b. 3%-5%
   c. 5%-10%
   d. 10%-12%

Reproductive System Concerns, Contraception, and Infertility

Reading Assignment: Contraception, Abortion, and Infertility (Chapter 4)

Patient: Maggie Gardner, Room 204

Goal: Demonstrate an understanding of reproductive system issues, contraception options, and infertility.

Objectives:

- Identify reproductive issues that can occur.
- Identify various methods of testing and treatment options that can be used for couples experiencing infertility.

Exercise 1

Writing Activity

5 minutes

1. _____% of the reproductive-age population has a problem with infertility.

2. The incidence of infertility increases in women at the age of _____.

3. List factors that affect female fertility.

4. List factors that affect male fertility.

Exercise 2

 CD-ROM Activity

 15 minutes

- Sign in to work at Pacific View Regional Hospital on the Obstetrics Floor for Period of Care 1. (*Note*: If you are already in the virtual hospital from a previous exercise, click on **Leave the Floor** and then on **Restart the Program** to get to the sign-in window.)
- From the Patient List, select Maggie Gardner (Room 204).
- Click on **Go to Nurses' Station**.
- Click on **Chart** and then on **204**.
- Click on **History and Physical** and review.

1. Maggie Gardner was married _____ years before she conceived.

2. Identify two factors that may have contributed to Maggie Gardner's inability to conceive for an extended period of time.

 3. With which of the following would Maggie Gardner have been diagnosed if she had chosen to get treatment after a year of attempting to get pregnant? (*Hint:* See pages 121-126 in your textbook.)
   a. Primary infertility
   b. Secondary infertility
   c. Tertiary infertility
   d. Situational-based infertility

4. List four tests that can be completed on the female to determine the causes of infertility.

5. List two tests that can be completed on the male to determine the causes of infertility.

6. What test is used to assess a couple to determine adequacy of coital technique?

7. What methods are available to assist the infertile couple in getting pregnant?

8. What methods did Maggie Gardner and her husband use to help in getting pregnant? (*Hint:* Look at the OB history in the History and Physical.)

LESSON 5 ——————————————————

Nursing Care During Pregnancy

 Reading Assignment: Anatomy and Physiology of Pregnancy (Chapter 6)
Nursing Care of the Family During Pregnancy (Chapter 7)

Patients: Kelly Brady, Room 203
Maggie Gardner, Room 204
Laura Wilson, Room 206

Goal: Demonstrate an understanding of the nursing care provided to women during normal pregnancy.

Objectives:

- Identify common physical and psychological findings associated with each trimester of pregnancy.
- Describe differences in the normal pregnancy changes experienced by adolescent and older mothers.

Exercise 1

 Writing Activity

5 minutes

1. The physician has recorded that a patient is postdates. Based on your understanding, you recognize that the patient:
   a. is in the third trimester of pregnancy.
   b. has completed the 37th week of pregnancy.
   c. is at least 40 weeks gestation.
   d. has completed 42 weeks of pregnancy.

2. Match the pregnancy term with the correct definition.

   Term

   _____ Gravida

   _____ Gravidity

   _____ Parity

   _____ Nullipara

   _____ Nulligravida

   Definition

   a. The number of pregnancies in which the fetus has reached 20 weeks gestation when born

   b. A woman who is pregnant

   c. A woman who has never been pregnant

   d. Pregnancy

   e. A woman who has never completed a pregnancy beyond 20 weeks gestation

3. Both serum and urine pregnancy tests are considered _____ signs of pregnancy.

4. List four positive signs of pregnancy.

5. Match each of the following behaviors in the pregnant woman with the trimester of pregnancy in which it is most likely to occur.

   Behavior

   _____ Fantasizes about the fetus

   _____ Is more interested in relationships with her mother and other women who are or have been pregnant

   _____ Experiences emotional lability

   _____ Is ready to have the pregnancy end

   _____ Has ambivalent feelings

   _____ May experience increased sexual desire as a result of increased pelvic congestion

   _____ Realistically prepares for birth and parenting the child

   Trimester

   a. Second trimester

   b. Third trimester

   c. Throughout pregnancy

6. A pregnant woman reports her partner has gained weight and has begun to complain of pregnancy-like physical complaints such as nausea and vomiting. What term can be used to describe this phenomenon?
   a. Paternal transference syndrome
   b. Paternal sympathy syndrome
   c. Couvade syndrome
   d. Pregnancy role reversal syndrome

7. The nurse makes note that the husband of a pregnant woman is demonstrating behaviors consistent with the moratorium phase. What is the primary developmental task of this stage?

Exercise 2

 CD-ROM Activity

 30 minutes

- Sign in to work at Pacific View Regional Hospital on the Obstetrics Floor for Period of Care 1. (*Note:* If you are already in the virtual hospital from a previous exercise, click on **Leave the Floor** and then on **Restart the Program** to get to the sign-in window.)
- From the Patient List, select Maggie Gardner (Room 204).
- Click on **Go to Nurses' Station**.
- Click on **Chart** and then on **204**.
- Click on **Nursing Admission**.

1. Place an X next to each subjective presumptive sign of pregnancy that applies to Maggie Gardner, according to the Nursing Admission. Select all that apply.

   _____ Amenorrhea

   _____ Nausea, vomiting

   _____ Breast changes

   _____ Urinary frequency

   _____ Fatigue

   _____ Quickening

2. Maggie Gardner is gravida _____, para _____.

3. Which of the following terms can be used to describe Maggie Gardner? Select all that apply.

_____ Nulligravida

_____ Nullipara

_____ Multigravida

_____ Multipara

_____ Primigravida

➤ • Click on **Return to Nurses' Station**.
• Click on **204** at the bottom of the screen.
• Click on **Patient Care**.
• Perform a focused physical assessment by clicking on **Abdomen** and then on **Reproductive**.

4. What positive pregnancy sign is found in Maggie Gardner's abdominal assessment?

➤ • Click on **Chart** and then on **204**.
• Click on **Nursing Admission**.

5. What is recorded as Maggie Gardner's LMP?

6. Using Nägele's rule, calculate Maggie Gardner's EDB. Explain how you calculated this date.

7. What is Maggie Gardner's gestational age?

8. Maggie Gardner is in the _____ trimester of pregnancy.

Exercise 3

 CD-ROM Activity

 15 minutes

 Laura Wilson and Kelly Brady represent age extremes among women of childbearing age. Read the sections on adolescents and women older than 35 years on pages 227-230 in your textbook.

- Sign in to work at Pacific View Regional Hospital on the Obstetrics Floor for Period of Care 4. (*Note:* If you are already in the virtual hospital from a previous exercise, click on **Leave the Floor** and then on **Restart the Program** to get to the sign-in window.)
- From the Nurses' Station, click on **Chart** and then on **206** for Laura Wilson's chart. (*Remember:* You are not able to visit patients or administer medications during Period of Care 4. You are only able to review patients' records.)
- Click on **Nursing Admission**.

1. In the left column of the table below, list common characteristics of pregnant adolescents, based on your textbook reading. Now, based on your chart review, consider how Laura Wilson compares with this textbook profile of the pregnant adolescent. Complete the right column of the table by explaining how each of the textbook characteristics applies to Laura Wilson.

Textbook Characteristic	Laura Wilson

2. What is Laura Wilson's gestational age?

3. Laura Wilson is in the _____ trimester of pregnancy.

→ • Now click on **Return to Nurses' Station**.
  • Click on **Chart** and then on **203** for Kelly Brady's chart.
  • Click on **Nursing Admission** and review.

4. In the left column of the table below, list common characteristics of older primiparous women, according to your textbook. Then, based on your chart review, think about how Kelly Brady compares with this textbook profile of the older primiparous mother. Complete the right column of the table by explaining how each of the textbook characteristics applies to Kelly Brady.

Textbook Characteristic	Kelly Brady

Maternal and Fetal Nutrition, Including Assessment of Risk Factors in Pregnancy

 Reading Assignment: Maternal and Fetal Nutrition (Chapter 8)
Assessment for High Risk Pregnancy (Chapter 19)
Pregnancy at Risk: Preexisting Conditions (Chapter 20)

Patients: Dorothy Grant, Room 201
Stacey Crider, Room 202
Kelly Brady, Room 203
Maggie Gardner, Room 204
Gabriela Valenzuela, Room 205
Laura Wilson, Room 206

Goal: Demonstrate an understanding of the assessment of risk factors in pregnancy, including maternal and fetal nutritional aspects.

Objectives:

- Identify appropriate interventions for maintaining adequate maternal and fetal nutrition.
- Differentiate among the varying types of assessment techniques that can be used with low-risk and high-risk pregnancy patients.
- Identify various methods of testing that can be used in high-risk pregnancies.

Exercise 1

CD-ROM Activity

30 minutes

- Sign in to work at Pacific View Regional Hospital on the Obstetrics Floor for Period of Care 1. (*Note*: If you are already in the virtual hospital from a previous exercise, click on **Leave the Floor** and then on **Restart the Program** to get to the sign-in window.)
- From the Patient List, select Maggie Gardner (Room 204).
- Click on **Go to Nurses' Station**.
- Click on **Chart** and then on **204**.
- Click on **Laboratory Reports** and review Maggie Gardner's test results.
- Click on **Physician's Orders** and review the ordered plan of care.

Review anemia on pages 247-267 and 610-611 in the textbook.

1. What were Maggie Gardner's hemoglobin and hematocrit levels on admission?

→ • Click on **History and Physical** and review this record.

2. What puts Maggie Gardner at a greater risk for developing anemia than the average pregnancy patient? (*Hint*: Review the Genetic Screening section of her History and Physical.)

3. What complication do women with anemia experience at a higher rate than those without anemia?

4. What medication has been ordered that will aid in the management of Maggie Gardner's anemia?

5. What supplements may be recommended for women who are taking iron supplements in pregnancy? Select all that apply.

_____ Zinc

_____ Calcium

_____ Vitamin D

_____ Copper

_____ Magnesium

6. What percentage of pregnant women are affected by anemia?
   a. 5%
   b. 15%
   c. 20%
   d. 30%

7. Maggie Gardner's physician has ordered a _____ diet.

8. What are some good sources of iron that you could encourage Maggie Gardner to add to her diet?

9. Maggie Gardner has gained _____ pounds during the pregnancy.

10. Maggie Gardner is 1.7 meters tall and weighed 165 pounds before becoming pregnant. What is her BMI?
    a. 20.12
    b. 23.75
    c. 25.95
    d. 29.34

11. Based on Maggie Gardner's BMI, it is recommended that she gain _____ to _____ during the pregnancy.

12. With consideration to the gestation of her pregnancy, it is recommended that Maggie Gardner increase her daily caloric intake by _____ over her prepregnant state.
    a. 200 calories
    b. 340 calories
    c. 462 calories
    d. 475 calories

13. What is a normal hematocrit level for women who are pregnant?

14. What assessments need to be performed by the nurse at each visit specifically related to an anemia diagnosis?

15. Maggie Gardner is not taking iron supplementation at this time; however, list three things that you could teach her about iron supplementation.

Exercise 2

 CD-ROM Activity

 20 minutes

1. A high-risk pregnancy is one in which the life or health of _____ or

_____ is jeopardized by a _____ coincidental with or unique to pregnancy.

• Sign in to work at Pacific View Regional Hospital on the Obstetrics Floor for Period of Care 3. (*Note*: If you are already in the virtual hospital from a previous exercise, click on **Leave the Floor** and then on **Restart the Program** to get to the sign-in window.)
• From the Patient List, select all six patients to review.
• Click on **Go to Nurses' Station**.
• Click on **Chart** and then on **201** to open Dorothy Grant's chart.
• Click on **History and Physical**.
• Click on **Return to Nurses' Station** and repeat the above steps for each patient until you have completed question 2.

2. Based on your chart review, list the factors that place each of these patients' pregnancies at risk.

Dorothy Grant

Stacey Crider

Kelly Brady

Maggie Gardner

Gabriela Valenzuela

Laura Wilson

3. A patient who consumes large amounts of caffeine may give birth to a newborn with a slight

   decrease in _____.

4. The exact effects of alcohol in pregnancy are not known. However, it can result in

   _____,

   _____, and

   _____.

5. Young mothers (under 15 years old) have a _____ higher mortality rate than those
   older than 20 years.

6. _____ occur in higher incidence with the first birth.

7. African-American babies have the highest rates of _____ and

   _____. The infant mortality rates among African

   Americans are more than _____ that of Caucasian rates.

Exercise 3

 CD-ROM Activity

 20 minutes

 1. List three things that ultrasounds are used for. (*Hint:* See pages 564-569 in your textbook.)

2. What are two forms of ultrasound, and when are they used?

 • Sign in to work at Pacific View Regional Hospital on the Obstetrics Floor for Period of Care 3. (*Note:* If you are already in the virtual hospital from a previous exercise, click on **Leave the Floor** and then on **Restart the Program** to get to the sign-in window.)
• From the Patient List, select Maggie Gardner (Room 204).
• Click on **Go to Nurses' Station**.
• Click on **Chart** and then on **204** for Maggie Gardner's chart.
• Click on the **Diagnostic Reports** and review the results.

3. What type of ultrasound is Maggie Gardner having?

4. Based on the ultrasound findings, how large is her baby?

5. List three abnormalities found on Maggie Gardner's ultrasound in regard to the placenta.

6. What is the impression from Maggie Gardner's ultrasound in terms of the fetus and the placenta?

7. What are the recommendations regarding follow-up?

Exercise 4

 CD-ROM Activity

 20 minutes

Biophysical profile is another very important assessment tool used with patients who are experiencing a high-risk pregnancy.

1. What are the five items that are assessed on a biophysical profile?

2. Abnormalities in the amniotic fluid index are frequently associated with

   _____.

3. The biophysical profile is an accurate indicator of impending _____.

4. The normal score on a biophysical profile is _____.

→ • Sign in to work at Pacific View Regional Hospital on the Obstetrics Floor for Period of
   Care 3. (*Note*: If you are already in the virtual hospital from a previous exercise, click on
   Leave the Floor and then on **Restart the Program** to get to the sign-in window.)
 • From the Patient List, select Kelly Brady (Room 203).
 • Click on **Go to Nurses' Station**.
 • Click on **Chart** and then on **203** for Kelly Brady's chart.
 • Click on **Diagnostic Reports** and review the results.

5. What is the estimated gestational age of Kelly Brady's fetus?

6. What is the amniotic fluid index as indicated on the report?

7. How does this correlate with the normal index as listed in the textbook?

8. What is the score on Kelly Brady's biophysical profile?

9. Based on what you have learned through your review of the textbook, what does this score
   indicate?

LESSON **7**

Nursing Care During Labor and Birth

Reading Assignment: Nursing Care of the Family During Labor and Birth
(Chapter 12)

Patients: Dorothy Grant, Room 201
Gabriela Valenzuela, Room 205
Laura Wilson, Room 206

Goal: Demonstrate an understanding of the normal labor and birth process.

Objectives:

• Assess and identify signs and symptoms present in each phase of Stage I labor.
• Describe appropriate nursing care for a patient in Stage I labor.

Exercise 1

 Writing Activity

5 minutes

1. A nurse is using nitrazine paper to determine whether the membranes of a patient have ruptured. The presence of what color on the paper is consistent with this phenomena?
   a. Blue
   b. Red
   c. Black
   d. Purple

2. When performing the psychosocial assessment of a laboring patient, what observations should be made concerning her nonverbal behaviors?

3. When providing care to a laboring patient, the nurse must remember to encourage voiding every _____ hours.
   a. 2
   b. 3
   c. 4
   d. 5

4. When a laboring woman is in bed, she should be assisted to change positions every _____ to _____ minutes.

5. A nurse is assisting a laboring patient into a semirecumbent position. The nurse recognizes that this position is beneficial for which of the following reasons?
   a. It will make performing back massage or applying counter pressure easier.
   b. It will facilitate internal rotation of the fetus.
   c. It reduces risk for perineal trauma.
   d. It is associated with less frequent, more intense contractions.

Exercise 2

 CD-ROM Activity

 20 minutes

- Sign in to work at Pacific View Regional Hospital on the Obstetrics Floor for Period of Care 1. (*Note*: If you are already in the virtual hospital from a previous exercise, click on **Leave the Floor** and then on **Restart the Program** to get to the sign-in window.)
- From the Patient List, select Dorothy Grant (Room 201).
- Click on **Go to Nurses' Station**.
- Click on **Chart** and then on **201** for Dorothy Grant's chart.
- Click on **Nurse's Notes**. Review the entry for Wednesday 0730.

1. List the findings from Dorothy Grant's most recent cervical exam.

→ • Click on **Return to Nurses' Station**.
  • Click on **EPR** and then on **Login**.
  • Select **201** from the Patient drop-down menu and **Obstetrics** from the Category drop-down menu.

2. At 0700, what was the recorded frequency and duration of Dorothy Grant's contractions?

→ • Now select **Vital Signs** from the Category drop-down menu.

3. At 0700, what was Dorothy Grant's recorded pain level?

4. At this time, in which phase of Stage I labor is Dorothy Grant? (*Hint:* Consult Table 12-1 in your textbook.)

5. Based on your review of the textbook and the patient's EPR, complete the table below and on the next page to compare typical findings for latent labor and Dorothy Grant's current condition.

Assessment	Typical Patient Findings	Dorothy Grant's Findings
Cervical dilation		
Contraction frequency		

Assessment	Typical Patient Findings	Dorothy Grant's Findings
Contraction duration		
Contraction intensity		

6. List the typical behaviors in latent phase labor.

→ • Click on **Exit EPR**.
  • Click on **201** at the bottom of the screen.
  • Click on **Patient Care** and then on **Nurse-Client Interactions**.
  • Select and view the video titled **0810: Monitoring/Patient Support**. (*Note:* Check the virtual clock to see whether enough time has elapsed. You can use the fast-forward feature to advance the time by 2-minute intervals if the video is not yet available. Then click again on **Patient Care** and **Nurse-Client Interactions** to refresh the screen.)

7. Based on the video interaction you just observed, place an X next to each characteristic that is true of Dorothy Grant. Select all that apply.

_____ Excited

_____ Thoughts center on self, labor, and baby

_____ Some apprehension

_____ Pain controlled fairly well

_____ Alert

_____ Follows directions readily

_____ Open to instructions

8. What interventions can be implemented to promote relaxation for Dorothy Grant during this phase of labor?

Exercise 3

 CD-ROM Activity

30 minutes

- Sign in to work at Pacific View Regional Hospital on the Obstetrics Floor for Period of Care 2. (*Note:* If you are already in the virtual hospital from a previous exercise, click on **Leave the Floor** and then on **Restart the Program** to get to the sign-in window.)
- From the Patient List, select Gabriela Valenzuela (Room 205).
- Click on **Go to Nurses' Station**.
- Click on **Chart** and then on **205**.
- Click on **Nurse's Notes**.
- Scroll down to review the entry for Wednesday 0800.

1. What was Gabriela Valenzuela's condition at 0800? What phase of labor was she experiencing?

2. As Gabriela Valenzuela progresses in labor, which phase will she enter next?

3. List common actions for the nurse or support person during active phase labor.

➔ • Still in the **Nurse's Notes**, scroll to the entry for Wednesday 1140. (*Note:* Check the virtual clock to see whether enough time has elapsed. You can use the fast-forward feature to advance the time by 2-minute intervals if the note is not yet available. Then exit and reenter the **Nurse's Notes** to refresh the screen.)

4. How is Gabriela Valenzuela tolerating labor at this time? Do you believe she has entered the active phase?

5. What assessments could be used to determine for certain which phase of labor Gabriela Valenzuela is currently experiencing?

• Click on **Return to Nurses' Station**.
 • Click on **205** at the bottom of the screen.
 • Click on **Patient Care** and then on **Nurse-Client Interactions**.
 • Select and view the video titled **1140: Intervention—Bleeding, Comfort**. (*Note:* Check the virtual clock to see whether enough time has elapsed. You can use the fast-forward feature to advance the time by 2-minute intervals if the video is not yet available. Then click again on **Patient Care** and **Nurse-Client Interactions** to refresh the screen.)

6. Based on the video interaction, place an X next to each intervention suggested or implemented by the nurse. Select all that apply.

_____ Limit assessment techniques to the time between contractions

_____ Help patient cope with contractions

_____ Encourage patient to help her maintain breathing techniques

_____ Use comfort measures

_____ Encourage voluntary muscle relaxation and use of effleurage

_____ Apply counter pressure to sacrococcygeal area

_____ Offer encouragement and praise

_____ Keep patient aware of progress

_____ Offer analgesics as ordered

_____ Check bladder; encourage voiding

_____ Give oral care; offer fluids, food, ice chips as ordered

 • Click on **Patient Care** and then on **Nurse-Client Interactions**.
 • Select and view the video titled **1155: Evaluation—Comfort Measures**. (*Note:* Check the virtual clock to see whether enough time has elapsed. You can use the fast-forward feature to advance the time by 2-minute intervals if the video is not yet available. Then click again on **Patient Care** and **Nurse-Client Interactions** to refresh the screen.)

7. Based on the video interaction, place an X next to each intervention suggested or implemented by the nurse and/or Gabriela Valenzuela's husband. Select all that apply.

_____ Limit assessment techniques to the time between contractions

_____ Help patient cope with contractions

_____ Encourage patient to help her maintain breathing techniques

_____ Use comfort measures

_____ Assist with position changes

_____ Encourage voluntary muscle relaxation and use of effleurage

_____ Apply counter pressure to sacrococcygeal area

_____ Offer encouragement and praise

_____ Keep patient aware of progress

_____ Offer analgesics as ordered

_____ Check bladder; encourage voiding

_____ Give oral care; offer fluids, food, ice chips as ordered

Exercise 4

 CD-ROM Activity

 30 minutes

- Sign in to work at Pacific View Regional Hospital on the Obstetrics Floor for Period of Care 4. (*Note:* If you are already in the virtual hospital from a previous exercise, click on **Leave the Floor** and then on **Restart the Program** to get to the sign-in window.)
- From the Nurses' Station, click on **EPR** and then on **Login**. (*Remember:* You are not able to visit patients or administer medications during Period of Care 4. You only are able to review patients' records.)
- In the Patient drop-down menu, select **201** for Dorothy Grant's records. Select **Obstetrics** from the Category drop-down menu.
- Scroll to review the entries for Wednesday 1800 and 1815.

1. What are the findings from Dorothy Grant's cervical exam at 1815?

2. At this time, which phase of Stage I labor is Dorothy Grant experiencing?

3. Complete the table below, listing typical findings for each assessment in the transition phase of Stage I labor.

Assessment	Typical Findings
Cervical dilation	
Contraction frequency	
Contraction duration	
Contraction intensity	

4. List the typical behaviors seen in patients experiencing the transition phase of labor.

→ • Click on **Exit EPR**.
  • Click on **Chart** and then on **201** for Dorothy Grant's chart.
  • Click on **Nurse's Notes**.
  • Read the notes recorded at 1800, 1815, and 1830 on Wednesday.

5. Based on information recorded in the EPR and Nurse's Notes, place an X next to each behavior Dorothy Grant exhibited during the transition phase of labor. Select all that apply.

_____ Severe pain

_____ Frustration; fear of loss of control

_____ Writhing with contractions

_____ Nausea/vomiting

_____ Perspiration

_____ Shaking or tremors

_____ Feeling of need to defecate

Now let's review Laura Wilson's status.

 • Click on **Return to Nurses' Station**.
• Click on **EPR** and then on **Login**.
• Select **206** from the Patient drop-down menu and **Vital Signs** from the Category drop-down menu.

6. Below, record Laura Wilson's assessment findings from 1815 on Wednesday.

Pain location

Pain intensity

 • Still in the EPR, select **Obstetrics** from the Category drop-down menu.

7. Below, record Laura Wilson's 1830 assessment findings.

Contraction frequency

Contraction duration

 • Now scroll back through earlier Obstetrics entries until you locate the results of Laura Wilson's most recent cervical exam.

8. When was Laura Wilson's most recent cervical examination performed? What were the results?

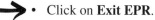 • Click on **Exit EPR**.
• Click on **Chart** and then on **206** for Laura Wilson's chart.
• Click on **Nurse's Notes**.
• Scroll to the note for Wednesday 1830.

9. According to this note, what event occurred at 1815?

10. List the immediate nursing actions appropriate for the situation you identified in question 9.

11. According to the Nurse's Notes and your textbook recommendations, did Laura Wilson's nurse handle this situation appropriately?

12. Based only on the information you have learned about Laura Wilson during this exercise, write the nursing diagnosis that you consider to be of highest priority for her at this time.

13. List several nursing interventions for the nursing diagnosis you wrote in question 12.

LESSON 8

Management of Discomfort

 Reading Assignment: Management of Discomfort (Chapter 10)

Patients: Kelly Brady, Room 203
Gabriela Valenzuela, Room 205
Laura Wilson, Room 206

Goal: Demonstrate an understanding of the normal labor and birth process.

Objectives:

- Assess and identify factors that influence pain perception.
- Describe selected nonpharmacologic and pharmacologic measures for pain management during labor and birth.

Exercise 1

 CD-ROM Activity

30 minutes

- Sign in to work at Pacific View Regional Hospital on the Obstetrics Floor for Period of Care 1. (*Note*: If you are already in the virtual hospital from a previous exercise, click on **Leave the Floor** and then on **Restart the Program** to get to the sign-in window.)
- From the Patient List, select Laura Wilson (Room 206).
- Click on **Get Report**.

1. What is Laura Wilson's condition when you assume care for her, according to the change-of-shift report?

• Click on **Go to Nurses' Station**.
 • Click on **206** at the bottom of the screen.
 • Read the **Initial Observations**.

2. What is your impression of Laura Wilson's condition?

 • Click on **Patient Care** and then on **Nurse-Client Interactions**.
 • Select and view the video titled **0730: Patient Assessment**. (*Note:* Check the virtual clock to see whether enough time has elapsed. You can use the fast-forward feature to advance the time by 2-minute intervals if the video is not yet available. Then click again on **Patient Care** and **Nurse-Client Interactions** to refresh the screen.)

3. What is Laura Wilson's assessment of her current condition? How does this compare with the information you received from the shift report and the Initial Observations summary?

 • Click on **Chart** and then on **206**.
 • Click on **Nursing Admission**.

4. List Laura Wilson's admission diagnoses. (*Hint:* See page 1 of the Nursing Admission form.)

5. What is your perception of Laura Wilson's behavior? What data did you collect during this exercise that led you to this perception?

6. Think about the following questions and then discuss your ideas with your classmates: Do your personal values and beliefs contribute to your perception of Laura Wilson's behavior? If so, how? What nursing interventions might help to overcome your personal biases when dealing with Laura Wilson?

• Continue reviewing Laura Wilson's Nursing Admission form as needed to answer question 7.

7. Each woman's pain during childbirth is unique and is influenced by a variety of factors. For each factor listed below, explain how that factor influences pain perception (in the middle column). Then, in the right column, list data from Laura Wilson's Nursing Admission that support how that factor might relate to her particular pain perception.

Factor	Typical Effect on Pain Perception	Laura Wilson's Supporting Data
Anxiety		
Previous experience		
Childbirth preparation		
Support		

Exercise 2

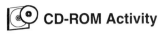 **CD-ROM Activity**

 45 minutes

- Sign in to work at Pacific View Regional Hospital on the Obstetrics Floor for Period of Care 2. (*Note*: If you are already in the virtual hospital from a previous exercise, click on **Leave the Floor** and then on **Restart the Program** to get to the sign-in window.)
- From the Patient List, select Gabriela Valenzuela (Room 205).

1. Focusing and relaxation techniques allow a woman in labor to rest and conserve energy by

   _____. While focusing on an object during a

   contraction, the woman _____ to reduce her

   _____ of pain. Varying breathing techniques are used to provide

   _____. All patterns begin and end with a _____.

2. Touch can communicate _____, _____, and

   _____. When using touch, it is important to determine the

   _____. Head, hand, back, and foot massage may

   be very effective in _____ and

   _____.

→ • Click on **Get Report**.

3. Is Gabriela Valenzuela in labor at this time? Give a rationale for your answer.

• Click on **Go to Nurses' Station**.
- Click on **205** at the bottom of the screen.
- Click on **Patient Care** and then on **Nurse-Client Interactions**.
- Select and view the video titled **1140: Intervention—Bleeding, Comfort**. (*Note:* Check the virtual clock to see whether enough time has elapsed. You can use the fast-forward feature to advance the time by 2-minute intervals if the video is not yet available. Then click again on **Patient Care** and **Nurse-Client Interactions** to refresh the screen.)
- Click on **Chart** and then on **205**.
- Click on **Nurse's Notes**.
- Scroll to the entry for 1140 on Wednesday. (*Note:* Check the virtual clock to see whether enough time has elapsed. You can use the fast-forward feature to advance the time by 2-minute intervals if the video is not yet available. Then click again on **Patient Care** and **Nurse-Client Interactions** to refresh the screen.)

4. How is Gabriela Valenzuela tolerating labor at this time?

5. Which of the following terms best describes the type of pain being experienced by Gabriela Valenzuela?
   a. Visceral
   b. Somatic
   c. Neuropathic
   d. Parasympathetic

6. What pain interventions does the nurse implement at this time?

7. What is the action of the fentanyl?

Let's begin the process for preparing and administering Gabriela Valenzuela's fentanyl dose.

 • Click on **Return to Nurses' Station**.
- Click on **MAR** and then on tab **205**.
- Scroll down to the PRN Medication Administration Record for Wednesday.

8. What is the ordered dose of fentanyl?

9. How long can the nurse expect the fentanyl to provide pain relief for Gabriela Valenzuela?
   a. 15-30 minutes
   b. 30 minutes-1 hour
   c. 1-2 hours
   d. 2-4 hours

10. Which of the following statements associated with fentanyl should the nurse understand when administering this medication to women in labor?

   _____ Fentanyl is distributed in the breast milk.

   _____ Fentanyl does not cross the placental barrier.

   _____ Fentanyl may prolong the latent stage of labor.

   _____ Fentanyl may facilitate cervical dilation when administered in the latent stage of labor.

→ • Click on **Return to Nurses' Station**.
   • Click on **Medication Room** at the bottom of the screen.
   • Click on **Automated System**.
   • Click on **Login**.
   • In box 1, click on **Gabriela Valenzuela, 205**.
   • In box 2, click on **Automated System Drawer A-F**.
   • Click on **Open Drawer**.
   • Click on **Fentanyl citrate**.
   • Click on **Put Medication on Tray**.
   • Click on **Close Drawer** at the bottom of the screen.
   • Click on **View Medication Room** at the bottom of the screen.
   • Click on **Preparation**.
   • Click on **Prepare** next to Fentanyl citrate and follow the Preparation Wizard prompts to prepare Gabriela Valenzuela's fentanyl dose. When the Wizard stops requesting information, click **Finish**.
   • Click on **Return to Medication Room** at the bottom of the screen.
   • Click on **205** at the bottom of the screen to go to the patient's room.

11. What additional assessments must be completed before you give Gabriela Valenzuela's medication?

12. Why is it important to check Gabriela Valenzuela's respirations before giving the dose of fentanyl?

13. What safety precautions should be in effect for Gabriela Valenzuela after she receives this dose of fentanyl?

 • Inside the patient's room, click on **Patient Care** and then on **Medication Administration**.
- Click on **Review Your Medications**. Click on the **Prepared** tab and verify the accuracy of your preparation. Then click **Return to Room 205**.
- Next, click the down arrow next to **Select** and choose to **Administer** the fentanyl citrate.
- Follow the Administration Wizard prompts to administer Gabriela Valenzuela's fentanyl dose. (*Note:* Click **Yes** when asked whether to document this administration in the MAR.)
- When the Wizard stops asking questions, click **Finish**.
- Still in Gabriela Valenzuela's room, click on **Patient Care** and then **Nurse-Client Interactions**.
- Select and view the video titled **1155: Evaluation—Comfort Measures**. (*Note:* Check the virtual clock to see whether enough time has elapsed. You can use the fast-forward feature to advance the time by 2-minute intervals if the video is not yet available. Then click again on **Patient Care** and **Nurse-Client Interactions** to refresh the screen.)

14. Based on the video interactions, how effective has the pain medication been?

15. Which of the following terms can be used to describe what Gabriela Valenzuela is experiencing? Select all that apply.

_____ Hyporespiration

_____ Hyperventilation

_____ Respiratory alkalosis

_____ Metabolic acidosis

_____ Orthostatic hypotension

16. What interventions does the nurse suggest to deal with this problem? List other interventions described in your textbook.

17. What could you tell Gabriela Valenzuela to help her make an informed decision about anesthesia for labor? Below, list advantages and disadvantages of epidural anesthesia.

Advantages   **Disadvantages**

Before leaving this period of care, let's see how you did preparing and administering the patient's medication.

- Click on **Leave the Floor**.
- Click on **Look at Your Preceptor's Evaluation**.
- Click on **Medication Scorecard** and review the evaluation. How did you do?
- Click on **Return to Evaluations**.
- Click on **Return to Menu**.

Exercise 3

 CD-ROM Activity

 15 minutes

- Sign in to work at Pacific View Regional Hospital on the Obstetrics Floor for Period of Care 4. (*Note*: If you are already in the virtual hospital from a previous exercise, click on **Leave the Floor** and then on **Restart the Program** to get to the sign-in window.)
- From the Nurses' Station, click on **Chart** and then on **203** for Kelly Brady's chart. (*Remember*: You are not able to visit patients or administer medications during Period of Care 4. You are only able to review patients' records.)
- Click on **Nurse's Notes**.
- Scroll to the entry for 1730 on Wednesday.

 Read the sections on Contraindications to Epidural Blocks and General Anesthesia on pages 306-307 in your textbook.

1. Why does the anesthesiologist plan to use general anesthesia during Kelly Brady's cesarean section?

2. Why is Kelly Brady upset about receiving general anesthesia for her surgery?

 • Click on **Physician's Orders**.
- Review the entry for Wednesday at 1540.

3. What preoperative medications were ordered for Kelly Brady?

 • Click on **Return to Nurses' Station**.
   • Click on the **Drug** icon in the lower left corner of your screen to access the Drug Guide.
   • Use the Search box or the scroll bar to read about each of the drugs you listed in question 3.

4. All of these medications are given preoperatively to help prevent aspiration pneumonia. Using information from the Drug Guide and from the section on General Anesthesia in your textbook, match each of the medications listed below with the description of how it specifically works to prevent aspiration pneumonia.

Medication	**Mechanism**
_____ Sodium citrate/citric acid (Bicitra)	a. Decreases the production of gastric acid
_____ Metoclopramide (Reglan)	b. Prevents nausea and vomiting and accelerates gastric emptying
_____ Ranitidine (Zantac)	c. Neutralizes acidic stomach contents

5. During general anesthesia, a short-acting barbiturate is administered to

   _____. A muscle relaxant is then

   given to _____. A low concentra-

   tion of a volatile halogenated agent may be administered to

   _____.

6. How would you expect general anesthesia to affect Kelly Brady's baby? Why?

9

Pregnancy at Risk: Gestational Diabetes Mellitus

🐍 **Reading Assignment:** Pregnancy at Risk: Preexisting Conditions (Chapter 20)

Patient: Stacey Crider, Room 202

Goal: Demonstrate an understanding of the identification and management of gestational diabetes mellitus (GDM).

Objectives:

- Identify appropriate interventions for controlling hyperglycemia in a patient with GDM.
- Correctly administer insulin to a patient with GDM.
- Plan and evaluate essential teaching for a patient with GDM.

Exercise 1

 CD-ROM Activity

 30 minutes

- Sign in to work at Pacific View Regional Hospital on the Obstetrics Floor for Period of Care 2. (*Note*: If you are already in the virtual hospital from a previous exercise, click on **Leave the Floor** and then on **Restart the Program** to get to the sign-in window.)
- From the Patient List, select Stacey Crider (Room 202).
- Click on **Go to Nurses' Station**.
- Click on **Chart** and then on **202**.
- Click on **History and Physical** and **Nursing Admission**.

1. Why has Stacey Crider been admitted to the hospital?

2. Stacey Crider is _____ weeks gestation.

3. When was Stacey Crider's GDM diagnosed? How has it been managed thus far?

4. Which of the following classifications is most characteristic of Stacey Crider's GDM?
   a. Class A1
   b. Class A2
   c. Class C
   d. Class C2

5. Read about risk factors for GDM on page 597 in your textbook. List these factors below.

- Search for evidence of the risk factors for GDM in Stacey Crider in the **History and Physical** and **Admissions** sections of her chart.

6. Which risk factors for GDM are present in Stacey Crider?

7. What does Stacey Crider's physician suspect is the cause of her poorly controlled blood glucose levels? (*Hint*: See the Impression section at the end of the History and Physical.)

→ • Click on **Physician's Orders**.

8. Find and review Stacey Crider's admission orders. Write down the orders that have been given to manage her GDM.

9. Why did Stacey Crider's physician order a hemoglobin A_{1C} test as part of her admission labs? (*Hint*: See page 586 in your textbook.)

10. What can be inferred from Stacey Crider's hemoglobin A_{1C} results?

On admission, Stacey Crider was in preterm labor. This was treated with magnesium sulfate tocolysis. She was also given a course of betamethasone.

→ • Click on **Return to Nurses' Station**.
  • Click on the **Drug** icon in the lower left corner of the screen.
  • Use the Search box or scroll down the drug list to find the entry for betamethasone.

11. How might betamethasone affect Stacey Crider's GDM?

→ • Click on **Return to Nurses' Station**.
  • Click on **Chart** and then on **202**.
  • Click on **Physician's Notes**.
  • Scroll to the note for Tuesday at 0700.

12. How does Stacey Crider's physician plan to deal with these potential medication effects?

Stacey Crider's other admission diagnosis is bacterial vaginosis (BV).

→ • Click on **Return to Nurses' Station**.
  • Click on **202** at the bottom of your screen.
  • Click on **Patient Care** and then on **Nurse-Client Interactions**.
  • Select and view the video titled **1115: Teaching—Diet, Infection**. (*Note:* Check the virtual clock to see whether enough time has elapsed. You can use the fast-forward feature to advance the time by 2-minute intervals if the video is not yet available. Then click again on **Patient Care** and **Nurse-Client Interactions** to refresh the screen.)

13. What is the relationship between Stacey Crider's bacterial vaginosis infection and her GDM?

Exercise 2

 CD-ROM Activity

 20 minutes

- Sign in to work at Pacific View Regional Hospital on the Obstetrics Floor for Period of Care 1. (*Note*: If you are already in the virtual hospital from a previous exercise, click on **Leave the Floor** and then on **Restart the Program** to get to the sign-in window.)
- From the Patient List, select Stacey Crider (Room 202).
- Click on **Go to Nurses' Station**.

 Stacey Crider needs her insulin so that she can eat breakfast. Recall that she receives lispro insulin prior to each meal and NPH insulin at bedtime. Read about the differences in these two types of insulin on pages 591-593 in your textbook.

1. Based on your textbook reading, complete the table below. (*Note*: NPH is considered an intermediate-acting insulin.)

Type of Insulin	Onset of Action	Peak	Duration
Lispro			
Intermediate-acting			

- Click on **EPR** and then on **Login**.
- Click on **202** in Patient drop-down menu. Select **Vital Signs** from the Category drop-down menu.
- Look at the vital sign assessment documented on Wednesday at 0700.

2. What is Stacey Crider's blood glucose?

→ • Click on **Exit EPR**.
  • Click on **MAR**.
  • Click on tab **202**.

3. What is Stacey Crider's prescribed insulin dosage?

→ • Click on **Return to Nurses' Station**.
  • Click on **Chart**.
  • Click on **202**.
  • Click on **Physician's Orders**.
  • Scroll to the orders for Tuesday at 1900.

4. How much insulin should Stacey Crider receive? Why?

→ • Click on **Return to Nurses' Station**.
  • Click on **Medication Room** at the bottom of the screen.
  • Click on **Unit Dosage**.
  • Click on drawer **202**.
  • Click on **Insulin Lispro**.
  • Click on **Put Medication on Tray**.
  • Click on **Close Drawer**.
  • Click on **View Medication Room**.
  • Click on **Preparation**.
  • Click on **Prepare** and follow the prompts to prepare Stacey Crider's lispro insulin dose.
  • Click on **Return to Medication Room**.

You are almost ready to give Stacey Crider's insulin injection. However, before you do . . .

5. Considering lispro insulin's rapid onset of action, what else should you check before giving Stacey Crider her injection?

Now you're ready!

- Click on **202** at the bottom of the screen.
- Click on **Check Armband**.
- Click on **Patient Care**.
- Click on **Medication Administration**.
- **Insulin Lispro** should be listed on the left side of your screen. Click on the down arrow next to **Select** and choose to **Administer** the insulin lispro.
- Follow the prompts to administer Stacey Crider's insulin injection. Indicate **Yes** to document the injection in the MAR and then click **Finish**.
- Click on **Leave the Floor**.
- Click on **Look at Your Preceptor's Evaluation**.
- Click on **Medication Scorecard**. How did you do?
- Click on **Return to Evaluations**.
- Click on **Return to Menu**.

Exercise 3

 CD-ROM Activity

 20 minutes

- Sign in to work at Pacific View Regional Hospital on the Obstetrics Floor for Period of Care 3. (*Note:* If you are already in the virtual hospital from a previous exercise, click on **Leave the Floor** and then on **Restart the Program** to get to the sign-in window.)
- From the Patient List, select Stacey Crider (Room 202).
- Click on **Go to Nurses' Station**.
- Click on **Chart** and then on **202**.
- Click on **Patient Education**.

Stacey Crider will likely be discharged home soon. Review her Patient Education record to determine her learning needs in relation to GDM.

1. List the educational goals for Stacey Crider regarding GDM.

2. Which of Stacey Crider's educational goals would apply to all women with GDM?

→ • Click on **Nurse's Notes** and scroll to the note for 0600 Wednesday.

3. How did the nurse describe Stacey Crider's ability to give her own insulin injection at that time?

→ • Click again on **Patient Education**.

4. What teaching was done with this patient on Wednesday in regard to GDM?

→ • Click on **Nurse's Notes** and review the note for 1200 Wednesday.

5. Do you think today's initial teaching on insulin administration was effective? Support your answer using objective documentation from the nurse's note.

Use the information you have obtained from the Patient Education form and the Nurse's Notes to answer the following questions.

6. Stacey Crider needs to know all of the following information. Which topic(s) would you choose to work on with her during this period of care? Select all that apply.

_____ Verbalize appropriate food choices and portions

_____ Demonstrate good technique when self-administering insulin

_____ Demonstrate good technique with self-monitoring of blood glucose

_____ Recognize hyper- and hypoglycemia and how to treat each

7. Give a rationale for your answer to question 6.

8. Which topic do you think Stacey Crider would choose to work on during this period of care?

_____ Verbalize appropriate food choices and portions

_____ Demonstrate good technique when self-administering insulin

_____ Demonstrate good technique with self-monitoring of blood glucose

_____ Recognize hyper- and hypoglycemia and how to treat each

9. Give a rationale for your answer to question 8.

Read the section on Postpartum Care on page 599 in your textbook. Stacey Crider has a significant risk for developing glucose intolerance later in life.

10. What advice would you give Stacey Crider to reduce this risk?

11. After delivery, what medical follow-up would you advise for Stacey Crider?

12. Could Stacey Crider's GDM affect her baby after birth? Explain.

Pregnancy at Risk: Cardiac Disorders, Lupus

 Reading Assignment: Pregnancy at Risk: Preexisting Conditions (Chapter 20)

Patients: Maggie Gardner, Room 204
Gabriela Valenzuela, Room 205

Goal: Demonstrate an understanding of the identification and management of selected medical-surgical problems in pregnancy.

Objectives:

- Identify appropriate interventions for managing selected medical-surgical problems in pregnancy.
- Plan and evaluate essential patient education during the acute phase of diagnosis.

Exercise 1

 CD-ROM Activity

15 minutes

- Sign in to work at Pacific View Regional Hospital on the Obstetrics Floor for Period of Care 1. (*Note*: If you are already in the virtual hospital from a previous exercise, click on **Leave the Floor** and then on **Restart the Program** to get to the sign-in window.)
- From the Patient List, select Gabriela Valenzuela (room 205).
- Click on **Go to Nurses' Station**.
- Click on **Chart** and then on **205**.
- Click on **History and Physical**.

1. According to the textbook, 1% to 4% of pregnancies are complicated by heart disease. In the History and Physical for Gabriela Valenzuela, what does the physician note as her cardiac problem?

2. _____ Mitral valve disease is one of the most common causes of cardiac disease in pregnant women. (True/False)

3. According to the History and Physical, what cardiac symptoms does Gabriela Valenzuela exhibit now that she is pregnant?

4. Based on your textbook reading, why do pregnant women with cardiac disorders have problems during their pregnancies?

5. What abnormal assessment finding is noted in the History and Physical that would be associated with Gabriela Valenzuela's cardiac disorder?

Exercise 2

 CD-ROM Activity

 20 minutes

Autoimmune disorders encompass a wide variety of disorders that can be disruptive to the pregnancy process. Maggie Gardner has been admitted to rule out systemic lupus erythematosus (SLE). This exercise will explore the various aspects of this autoimmune disorder.

- Sign in to work at Pacific View Regional Hospital on the Obstetrics Floor for Period of Care 2. (*Note*: If you are already in the virtual hospital from a previous exercise, click on **Leave the Floor** and then on **Restart the Program** to get to the sign-in window.)
- From the Patient List, select Maggie Gardner (Room 204).
- Click on **Go to Nurses' Station**.
- Click on **Chart** and then on **204**.
- Click on **History and Physical**.

1. Based on your textbook reading, what information in Maggie Gardner's History and Physical would correlate to a diagnosis of SLE?

2. What are some early symptoms of SLE that are often overlooked?

➔ - Click on **Return to Nurses' Station**.
- Click on **204** at the bottom of the screen.
- Click on **Patient Care** and then on **Physical Assessment**.
- One at a time, click on the various body areas (yellow boxes) and system subcategories (green boxes) to complete a head-to-toe assessment of Maggie Gardner.

3. Based on your head-to-toe assessment, list four abnormal findings related to Maggie Gardner's diagnosis.

- Click on **Chart** and then on **204**.
- Click on **Patient Education**.

4. Based on your head-to-toe assessment, the information in the Patient Education section of the chart, and the fact that this is a new diagnosis for the patient, list three areas of teaching that need to be completed with Maggie Gardner.

Exercise 3

 CD-ROM Activity

 30 minutes

- Sign in to work at Pacific View Regional Hospital on the Obstetrics Floor for Period of Care 3. (*Note*: If you are already in the virtual hospital from a previous exercise, click on **Leave the Floor** and then on **Restart the Program** to get to the sign-in window.)
- From the Patient List, select Maggie Gardner (Room 204).
- Click on **Go to Nurses' Station**.
- Click on **Chart** and then on **204**.
- Click on the **Consultations** tab.
- Scroll down and review the Rheumatology Consult.

1. After the review of systems, list four things that the rheumatologist notes in the Impressions section of the consult regarding specific findings associated with Maggie Gardner's diagnosis of SLE.

→ • Now click on **Diagnostic Reports**.

2. Maggie Gardner had an ultrasound done prior to the consult with the rheumatologist. What were the findings as they would relate to SLE? What were the follow-up recommendations? (*Hint*: See Impressions section.)

3. What is the rheumatologist's plan regarding laboratory/diagnostics to gain a definitive diagnosis?

4. According to the consult, what is the plan regarding medications for Maggie Gardner (immediate need)?

• Click on **Return to Nurses' Station**.

• Click on the **Drug** icon in the lower left corner of the screen.

• Use the Search box or the scroll bar to find the entry for prednisone.

5. What does Maggie Gardner need to be taught regarding this medication?

 • Click on **Return to Nurses' Station**.

• Click on **204** at the bottom of the screen.

• Click on **Patient Care** and then on **Nurse-Client Interactions**.

• Select and view the video titled **1530: Disease Management**. (*Note:* Check the virtual clock to see whether enough time has elapsed. You can use the fast-forward feature to advance the time by 2-minute intervals if the video is not yet available. Then click again on **Patient Care** and **Nurse-Client Interactions** to refresh the screen.)

6. During this video, the nurse provides Maggie Gardner with information regarding her disease. What two things does the nurse note that are important aspects of managing this disease during pregnancy?

7. What medication ordered by the rheumatologist will assist in the blood flow to the placenta? How?

8. What key component does the nurse identify for Maggie Gardner that will assist in maintaining a healthy pregnancy?

9. What excuse does Maggie Gardner give for not keeping previous doctor's appointments? (*Hint:* This information is also found in the Nursing Admission in the chart.)

Exercise 4

 CD-ROM Activity

 20 minutes

- Sign in to work at Pacific View Regional Hospital on the Obstetrics Floor for Period of Care 4. (*Note:* If you are already in the virtual hospital from a previous exercise, click on **Leave the Floor** and then on **Restart the Program** to get to the sign-in window.)
- From the Nurses' Station, click on **Chart**. (*Remember:* You are not able to visit patients or administer medications during Period of Care 4. You are only able to review patients' records.)
- Click on **204** to open Maggie Gardner's chart.
- Click on **Laboratory Reports**.

1. Maggie Gardner's laboratory results for tests that were ordered during Period of Care 2 are now available. What are the findings?

Laboratory Test	Result
C3	
C4	
CH50	
RPR	
ANA titer	
Anticardiolipin	
Anti-sm; Anti-DNA; Anti–SSA	
Anti-SSB	
Anti-RVV; Antiphospholipid	

• Click on **Consultations** and scroll down to review the Rheumatology Consult.

2. The lab findings you recorded in question 1 are definitive for the diagnosis of SLE. According to the textbook and the Rheumatology Consult, what is the plan to manage this disease once Maggie Gardner's baby is delivered?

 • Click on **Nurse's Notes.**

3. By Period of Care 4, Maggie Gardner has been provided with education regarding various aspects of her disease process, testing, and hospital procedures. Based on your review of the Nurse's Notes for Wednesday, what has she been specifically taught? (Provide time and instruction provided.)

4. Using correct NANDA terminology, list three possible nursing diagnoses for Maggie Gardner.

5. SLE requires long-term management because patients will experience remissions and exacerbations. What step did the rheumatologist take with Maggie Gardner to begin the long-term relationship that will be required to ensure a healthy outcome? (*Hint:* Return to the Consultations section of the chart.)

Pregnancy at Risk: Severe Preeclampsia

 Reading Assignment: Pregnancy at Risk: Gestational Conditions (Chapter 21)

Patient: Kelly Brady, Room 203

Goal: Demonstrate an understanding of the identification and management of severe preeclampsia.

Objectives:

- Assess and identify signs and symptoms present in the patient with severe preeclampsia.
- Explain how common signs and symptoms present in the patient with severe preeclampsia relate to the underlying pathophysiology of this disease.
- Identify the patient who has developed HELLP syndrome.
- Describe routine nursing care for the patient with severe preeclampsia who is receiving magnesium sulfate.

Exercise 1

 CD-ROM Activity

30 minutes

- Sign in to work at Pacific View Regional Hospital on the Obstetrics Floor for Period of Care 3. (*Note:* If you are already in the virtual hospital from a previous exercise, click on **Leave the Floor** and then on **Restart the Program** to get to the sign-in window.)
- From the Patient List, select Kelly Brady (Room 203).
- Click on **Go to Nurses' Station**.
- Click on **Chart** and then on **203**.
- Click on **History and Physical**.

1. What was Kelly Brady's admission diagnosis?

2. Using the History and Physical and information from Table 21-2 in your textbook, complete the table below.

Sign/Symptom	Mild Preeclampsia	Severe Preeclampsia	Kelly Brady on Admission
Blood pressure			
Proteinuria			
Headache			
Reflexes			
Visual problems			
Epigastric pain			

3. Which of the following are risk factors for the development of preeclampsia? Select all that apply.

_____ Multiparity

_____ Family history of preeclampsia

_____ Obesity

_____ History of gestational diabetes

_____ Type 1 diabetes mellitus

_____ Renal disease

→ • Click on **Physician's Orders** and scroll down to find the admitting physician's orders on Tuesday at 1030.

4. What tests and/or procedures did Kelly Brady's physician order to confirm the diagnosis of severe preeclampsia?

→ • Click on **Physician's Notes**.
 • Scroll down to the note for Wednesday 0730.

5. What subjective and objective data are recorded here that would support the diagnosis of severe preeclampsia?

Kelly Brady's 24-hour urine collection was completed and sent to the lab at 1230.

→ • Click on **Laboratory Reports**.
 • Scroll to find the Wednesday 1230 results.

6. What were the results of Kelly Brady's 24-hour urine collection?

7. Now list all the data you have collected during this exercise that confirm Kelly Brady's diagnosis of severe preeclampsia.

Exercise 2

 CD-ROM Activity

 30 minutes

- Sign in to work at Pacific View Regional Hospital on the Obstetrics Floor for Period of Care 3. (*Note*: If you are already in the virtual hospital from a previous exercise, click on **Leave the Floor** and then on **Restart the Program** to get to the sign-in window.)
- From the Patient List, select Kelly Brady (Room 203).
- Click on **Go to Nurses' Station**.

1. Kelly Brady had blood drawn at 1230 for an AST measurement and a platelet count. Why do you think this was done?

 • Click on **Chart** and then on **203**.
- Click on **Laboratory Reports**.
- Scroll down to the report for Wednesday 1230 to locate the results of these tests.

2. Complete the table below based on your review of the Laboratory Reports and your textbook.

Test	Wed 1230 Result	Normal Nonpregnant Value	Value in HELLP
Platelet count			
AST			

→ • Click on **Return to Nurses' Station**.
  • Click on **Patient List**.
  • Click on **Get Report** for Kelly Brady.

3. Why has Kelly Brady been transferred to Labor and Delivery?

4. In addition to prematurity, what risk factors are associated with preeclampsia?

5. HELLP syndrome is not a separate illness, but a _____.

   However, many women with HELLP syndrome are _____ or have only

   slightly elevated blood pressure. HELLP syndrome consists of intravascular

   _____, _____ enzymes, and

   _____ count. HELLP syndrome is a _____

   diagnosis.

• Click on **Return to Nurses' Station**.
- Click on **Chart** and then on **203**.
- Click on **Physician's Notes**. (*Note:* Check the virtual clock to see whether enough time has elapsed. You can use the fast-forward feature to advance the time by 2-minute intervals if the video is not yet available. Then click again on **Patient Care** and **Nurse-Client Interactions** to refresh the screen.)
- Scroll to the note for Wednesday 1530.

6. What is the physician's plan of care for Kelly Brady, in light of the HELLP syndrome diagnosis?

7. All of the assessments/interventions listed below are part of routine nursing care for a patient with severe preeclampsia. Place an X next to each activity that is performed specifically to assess for magnesium toxicity. Select all that apply.

_____ Measure/record urine output

_____ Measure proteinuria using urine dipstick

_____ Monitor liver enzyme levels and platelet count

_____ Monitor for headache, visual disturbances, and epigastric pain

_____ Assess for decreased level of consciousness

_____ Assess DTRs

_____ Weigh daily to assess for edema

_____ Monitor vital signs, especially respiratory rate

_____ Dim room lights and maintain a quiet environment

Pregnancy at Risk: Antepartal Hemorrhagic Disorders

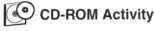 **Reading Assignment:** Pregnancy at Risk: Gestational Conditions (Chapter 21)

Patient: Gabriela Valenzuela, Room 205

Goal: Demonstrate an understanding of the identification and management of selected hemorrhagic complications of pregnancy.

Objectives:

- Identify appropriate interventions for managing abruptio placenta.
- Differentiate between the symptoms related to an abruptio placenta and those related to a placenta previa.
- Plan and evaluate essential patient education during the acute phase of diagnosis.

Exercise 1

 CD-ROM Activity

🕐 30 minutes

- Sign in to work at Pacific View Regional Hospital on the Obstetrics Floor for Period of Care 1. (*Note*: If you are already in the virtual hospital from a previous exercise, click on **Leave the Floor** and then on **Restart the Program** to get to the sign-in window.)
- From the Patient List, select Gabriela Valenzuela (Room 205).
- Click on **Go to Nurses' Station**.
- Click on **Chart** and then on **205**.
- Click on **Emergency Department**.

1. What transpired that brought Gabriela Valenzuela to the emergency department? How long did she wait before coming to the emergency department? What was the deciding factor in her coming to the emergency department?

2. In addition to a motor vehicle accident, what other factors could result in or increase the risk for having an abruptio placenta?

3. Differential diagnosis is very important when you are confronted with clinical manifestations that could be evidence of more than one process. Using your textbook as a guide, compare the characteristics and complications of abruptio placenta and placenta previa below.

Characteristic/Complication	Abruptio Placenta	Placenta Previa
Bleeding		
Shock complication		
Coagulopathy (DIC)		
Uterine tonicity		
Tenderness/pain		
Placenta findings		
Fetal effects		

4. Based on the Emergency Department report in her chart, what grade of abruption does Gabriela Valenzuela have? Provide supporting documentation from the textbook reading.

 • Click on **Return to Nurses' Station**.

• Click on **205** at the bottom of the screen to go to the patient's room.

• Click on the **Patient Care** and then **Nurse-Client Interactions**.

• Select and view the video titled **0740: Patient Teaching—Fetal Monitoring**. (*Note:* Check the virtual clock to see whether enough time has elapsed. You can use the fast-forward feature to advance the time by 2-minute intervals if the video is not yet available. Then click again on **Patient Care** and **Nurse-Client Interactions** to refresh the screen.)

5. Once Gabriela Valenzuela is admitted to the floor, what are her and her husband's concerns? What does the nurse include in her teaching to alleviate those concerns?

 • Next, select and view the video titled **0805: Patient Teaching—Abruption**. (*Note:* Check the virtual clock to see whether enough time has elapsed. You can use the fast-forward feature to advance the time by 2-minute intervals if the video is not yet available. Then click again on **Patient Care** and **Nurse-Client Interactions** to refresh the screen.)

6. What specific interventions will assist in increasing the oxygen supply to the baby and prevent further separation of the placenta?

Exercise 2

  CD-ROM Activity

25 minutes

- Sign in to work at Pacific View Regional Hospital on the Obstetrics Floor for Period of Care 1. (*Note*: If you are already in the virtual hospital from a previous exercise, click on **Leave the Floor** and then on **Restart the Program** to get to the sign-in window.)
- From the Patient List, select Gabriela Valenzuela (Room 205).
- Click on **Go to Nurses' Station**.

Gabriela Valenzuela is at increased risk for early delivery as a result of abdominal trauma and the subsequent occurrence of grade 1 abruptio placenta. She is currently manifesting signs and symptoms of early labor. According to the Emergency Department report, she was given a dose of betamethasone, which was to be repeated in 12 hours.

1. What is the purpose of the administration of betamethasone in this patient's scenario?

- Click on **MAR** and then on tab **205**.
- Review the betamethasone dosage to be given.
- Click on **Return to Nurses' Station**.
- Click on **Medication Room** at the bottom of the screen.
- Click on **Unit Dosage**.
- Click on drawer **205**.
- Click on **Betamethasone**.
- Click on **Put Medication on Tray**.
- Click on **Close Drawer**.
- Click on **View Medication Room**.
- Click on **Preparation**.
- Click on **Prepare** and follow the prompts to complete preparation of Gabriela Valenzuela's betamethasone.
- Click on **Return to Medication Room**.
- Click on **205** at the bottom of the screen.
- Click on **Patient Care**.
- Click on **Medication Administration**.
- Click on **Review Your Medications**.
- Click on the **Prepared** tab at the top of the screen.

2. According to the text box on the right, what is the medication name and dosage that you have prepared for Gabriela Valenzuela?

3. How many mg are you giving to Gabriela Valenzuela based on the answer to the previous question? Is this the correct dosage based on the MAR?

→ • Click on **Return to Room 205**.
 • Click on the **Drug** icon in the lower left corner of the screen to access the Drug Guide.
 • Use the Search box or scroll bar to find the entry for betamethasone.

4. Based on the information provided in the Drug Guide, what is the dosage for pregnant adults?

5. Based on your review of the baseline assessment data in the Drug Guide, what areas need to be assessed in Gabriela Valenzuela's history?

6. Still in the Drug Guide, review the information regarding the administration of this medication. What are three things that need to be taken into consideration when giving this medication in the injection form?

You are now ready to complete the medication administration.

- Click on **Return to Room 205**.
- Click on **Check Armband**.
- Click on the down arrow next to Select (to the right of betamethasone) and choose **Administer**.
- Follow the prompts to administer Gabriela Valenzuela's betamethasone. Document the administration in the MAR.
- Click on **Leave the Floor**.
- Click on **Look at Your Preceptor's Evaluation**.
- Click on **Medication Scorecard**. How did you do?
- Click on **Return to Evaluations**.
- Click on **Return to Menu**.

Exercise 3

 CD-ROM Activity

 25 minutes

- Sign in to work at Pacific View Regional Hospital on the Obstetrics Floor for Period of Care 2. (*Note*: If you are already in the virtual hospital from a previous exercise, click on **Leave the Floor** and then on **Restart the Program** to get to the sign-in window.)
- From the Patient List, select Gabriela Valenzuela (Room 205).
- Click on **Go to Nurses' Station**.
- Click on **Chart** and then on **205**.
- Click on **Diagnostic Reports**.

1. Gabriela Valenzuela had an ultrasound done on Tuesday to determine the source of her vaginal bleeding. What were the findings on the ultrasound?

- Click on the **Laboratory Reports**.

2. What were Gabriela Valenzuela's hemoglobin and hematocrit levels on Tuesday? How do these findings compare with Wednesday's report? Has there been a significant change?

3. According to the textbook information, the hematocrit level needs to be maintained at

   _____.

4. What findings are associated with a severe abruption?

 • Click on **Return to Nurses' Station**.
   • Click on **EPR** and then on **Login**.
   • Select **205** from the Patient drop-down menu and select **Vital Signs** from the category drop-down menu.
   • Using the right and left arrows, scroll to review the patient's vital signs over the last 12 hours.

5. From 0000 Wednesday until 1200 Wednesday, would you consider Gabriela Valenzuela's condition stable or unstable? State the rationale for your answer.

 • Click on **Exit EPR**.
   • Click on **205** at the bottom of the screen.
   • Click on **Patient Care** and then on **Nurse-Client Interactions**.
   • Select and view the video titled **1140: Intervention—Bleeding, Comfort**. Take notes as you watch and listen. (*Note:* Check the virtual clock to see whether enough time has elapsed. You can use the fast-forward feature to advance the time by 2-minute intervals if the video is not yet available. Then click again on **Patient Care** and **Nurse-Client Interactions** to refresh the screen.)

6. What happened that elicited this interaction? (*Hint*: Review the Nurse's Notes for 1140.)

7. What actions did the nurse take during the interaction?

Exercise 4

 CD-ROM Activity

 25 minutes

- Sign in to work at Pacific View Regional Hospital on the Obstetrics Floor for Period of Care 3. (*Note*: If you are already in the virtual hospital from a previous exercise, click on **Leave the Floor** and then on **Restart the Program** to get to the sign-in window.)
- From the Patient List, select Gabriela Valenzuela (Room 205).
- Click on **Go to Nurses' Station**.
- Click on **Kardex**.
- Click on tab **205**.

1. What problem areas have been identified by the nurse related to Gabriela Valenzuela's diagnosis?

2. What is the focus of the outcomes related to the above-mentioned problem areas?

3. Using correct NANDA terminology, list four possible nursing diagnoses appropriate for Gabriela Valenzuela.

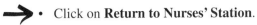 • Click on **Return to Nurses' Station**.
- Click on **Chart** and then on **205**.
- Click on **Patient Education**.

4. According to the patient education sheet in Gabriela Valenzuela's chart, what are the educational goals related to the patient's diagnosis?

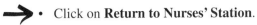 • Click on **Nurse's Notes**.

5. According to the Nurse's Notes, what education has been completed by the nurses through Period of Care 3? Include documentation of the times and topics.

6. What are some barriers to learning that the nurse may confront with this patient? (*Hint:* Review the Nurse's Notes.)

7. How can the nurse overcome each of these potential barriers?

LESSON 13

Labor and Birth at Risk

 Reading Assignment: Labor and Birth at Risk (Chapter 22)

Patients: Dorothy Grant, Room 201
Stacey Crider, Room 202
Kelly Brady, Room 203
Gabriela Valenzuela, Room 205

Goal: Demonstrate an understanding of the identification and management of selected labor and birth complications.

Objectives:

- Assess and identify signs and symptoms present in the patient with preterm labor.
- Describe appropriate nursing care for the patient in preterm labor.
- Develop a birth plan to meet the needs of the preterm infant.

Exercise 1

 CD-ROM Activity

20 minutes

- Sign in to work at Pacific View Regional Hospital on the Obstetrics Floor for Period of Care 2. (*Note*: If you are already in the virtual hospital from a previous exercise, click on **Leave the Floor** and then on **Restart the Program** to get to the sign-in window.)
- From the Patient List, select Dorothy Grant (Room 201) and Gabriela Valenzuela (Room 205).
- Click on **Go to Nurses' Station**.
- Click on **Chart** and then on **201** for Dorothy Grant's chart.
- Click on **History and Physical**.

1. Using the data from the History and Physical, complete the table below for Dorothy Grant.

Patient	Weeks Gestation	Reason for Admission
Dorothy Grant		

- Click on **Return to Nurses' Station**.
- Click again on **Chart**; this time, select **205** for Gabriela Valenzuela's chart.
- Click on **History and Physical**.

2. Using the data from the History and Physical, complete the table below for Gabriela Valenzuela.

Patient	Weeks Gestation	Reason for Admission
Gabriela Valenzuela		

- Click on **Return to Nurses' Station**.
- Click on **201** at the bottom of the screen to go to Dorothy Grant's room.
- Inside the patient's room, click on **Patient Care**.
- Click on **Physical Assessment**.
- Click on **Pelvic** and then on **Reproductive**.

3. Complete the table below with the results of Dorothy Grant's initial cervical examination.

Patient	Time	Dilation	Effacement	Station
Dorothy Grant				

- Click on **205** at the bottom of the screen to go to Gabriela Valenzuela's room.
- Click on **Patient Care**.
- Click on **Physical Assessment**.
- Click on **Pelvic** and then on **Reproductive**.

4. Record the results of Gabriela Valenzuela's initial cervical examination in the table below.

Patient	Time	Dilation	Effacement	Station
Gabriela Valenzuela				

5. What criteria are necessary in order to make a diagnosis of preterm labor?

6. As of Wednesday at 0800, would you consider either or both of these patients to be in preterm labor? Give a rationale for your answer.

 Read the section on tocolysis on pages 683-684 in your textbook to answer the following questions.

7. Would you recommend tocolytic therapy for Gabriela Valenzuela? Support your answer.

8. Match each of the medications below with the description of how it works as a tocolytic agent. (*Hint:* Answers may be used more than once.)

Medication	Tocolytic Mechanism
_____ Magnesium sulfate	a. Inhibits calcium from entering smooth muscle cells, thus reducing uterine contractions
_____ Nifedipine (Procardia)	
_____ Ritodrine (Yutopar)	b. Relaxes uterine smooth muscle as a result of stimulation of beta$_2$ receptors on uterine smooth muscle
_____ Terbutaline (Brethine)	
_____ Indomethacin (Indocin)	c. Exact mechanism unclear, but promotes relaxation of smooth muscles
	d. Suppresses preterm labor by blocking the production of prostaglandins

Exercise 2

 CD-ROM Activity

 30 minutes

- Sign in to work at Pacific View Regional Hospital on the Obstetrics Floor for Period of Care 1. (*Note*: If you are already in the virtual hospital from a previous exercise, click on **Leave the Floor** and then on **Restart the Program** to get to the sign-in window.)
- From the Patient List, select Dorothy Grant (Room 201), Stacey Crider (Room 202), and Kelly Brady (Room 203).
- Click on **Get Report** for Stacey Crider.

Stacey Crider was admitted yesterday in preterm labor and placed on magnesium sulfate. Her other admission diagnoses were bacterial vaginosis and gestational diabetes with poorly controlled blood glucose levels.

1. What is Stacey Crider's current status in regard to preterm labor?

- Click on **Go to Nurses' Station**.
- Click on **Chart** and then on **202** for Stacey Crider's chart.
- Click on **Physician's Orders**.
- Scroll down to the orders for Wednesday at 0715.

2. Which of these orders relates specifically to Stacey Crider's diagnosis of preterm labor?

→ • Scroll up to the orders for Wednesday at 0730.

3. What medication changes are ordered?

4. Why do you think Stacey Crider's physician changed his orders so quickly?

→ • Click on **Return to Nurses' Station**.
   • Click on **202** at the bottom of the screen.
   • Inside Stacey Crider's room, click on **Take Vital Signs**.

5. What are Stacey Crider's current vital signs?

   T

   HR

   RR

   BP

6. Which of the above parameters provides the most important information needed before giving Stacey Crider's nifedipine dose? Why? (*Hint*: Read about nifedipine on page 684 in your textbook.)

Like Dorothy Grant and Kelly Brady, Stacey Crider is also receiving betamethasone.

 Read about the promotion of fetal lung maturity on page 684 in your textbook; then answer the following questions.

7. Why are all three of these patients receiving antenatal glucocorticoid therapy?

 • Click on **MAR**.
   • Click on tab **202**.

8. What is Stacey Crider's prescribed betamethasone dosage?

 9. How does this dosage compare with the recommended dosage listed in the Antenatal Glucocorticoid Therapy Medication Guide on page 684 in the textbook?

 • Click on **Return to Room 202**.
   • Click on **Medication Room** at the bottom of the screen.
   • Click on **Unit Dosage**.
   • Click on drawer **202**.
   • Click on **Betamethasone**.
   • Click on **Put Medication on Tray**.
   • Click on **Close Drawer**.
   • Click on **View Medication Room**.
   • Click on **Preparation**.
   • Click on **Prepare** and follow the Preparation Wizard's prompts to complete preparation of Stacey Crider's betamethasone dose.
   • Click on **Return to Medication Room**.
   • Click on **202** at the bottom of the screen to return to Stacey Crider's room.

- Click on **Check Armband**.
- Click on **Check Allergies**.
- Click on **Patient Care**.
- Click on **Medication Administration**.
- Find **Betamethasone** listed on the left side of your screen. To its right, click on the down arrow next to **Select** and choose **Administer**.
- Follow the Administration Wizard's prompts to administer Stacey Crider's betamethasone injection. Indicate **Yes** to document the injection in the MAR and then click **Finish**.
- Click on **Leave the Floor**.
- Click on **Look at Your Preceptor's Evaluation**.
- Click on **Medication Scorecard** for Stacey Crider. How did you do?
- Click on **Return to Evaluations**.
- Click on **Return to Menu**.

Exercise 3

 CD-ROM Activity

 30 minutes

- Sign in to work at Pacific View Regional Hospital on the Obstetrics Floor for Period of Care 4. (*Note*: If you are already in the virtual hospital from a previous exercise, click on **Leave the Floor** and then on **Restart the Program** to get to the sign-in window.)
- Click on **Chart** and then **201** for Dorothy Grant's chart. (*Remember:* You are not able to visit patients or administer medications during Period of Care 4. You are only able to review patients' records only.)
- Click on **Nurse's Notes**.
- Scroll down to the note for Wednesday 1815.

1. Despite receiving terbutaline for tocolysis, Dorothy Grant's labor continues to progress. What are the findings from Dorothy Grant's cervical examination at this time?

 - Scroll up to the note for Wednesday 1840. It states that Dorothy Grant is being prepped for delivery.

2. If you were the nurse caring for Dorothy Grant during delivery, what special preparations would you make to care for the baby immediately after birth?

• Click on **Return to Nurses' Station**.
  • Click again on **Chart**, but this time choose **205** for Gabriela Valenzuela's chart.
  • Click on **Physician's Notes**.
  • Scroll down to the note for Wednesday 0800.

  3. What is the anticipated outcome of Gabriela Valenzuela's labor, according to this note?

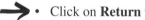 • Scroll up to the notes for 1415 and 1455.

  4. What preparations have been made during the day for the birth of Gabriela Valenzuela's baby?

 • Click on **Return to Nurses' Station**.
  • Once again, click on **Chart**; select **203** for Kelly Brady's chart.
  • Click on **Physician's Notes**.
  • Scroll down to the note for Wednesday 1530.

Kelly Brady was admitted yesterday with severe preeclampsia at 26 weeks gestation. Her preeclampsia is now worsening.

  5. Why does her physician now recommend immediate delivery?

6. What general risks related to cesarean section does Kelly Brady's physician discuss with her?

 7. Because of Kelly Brady's early gestational age (26 weeks), her physician anticipates a classical uterine incision. How will this type of incision affect Kelly Brady's birth options in future pregnancies? (*Hint:* Read the section on vaginal birth after cesarean on pages 713-714 in your textbook.)

 • Click on **Physician's Orders**.
  • Review the orders for 1540.

8. Below, list the orders to be carried out before Kelly Brady's surgery. State the purpose of each.

Order	Purpose

9. Can you think of other common preoperative procedures? List them below. (*Hint*: Refer to a basic Medical-Surgical textbook for ideas if you need help!)

LESSON 14

The Newborn at Risk

/☞ **Reading Assignment:** The Newborn at Risk (Chapter 24)

Patients: Stacey Crider, Room 202
Kelly Brady, Room 203
Gabriela Valenzuela, Room 205
Laura Wilson, Room 206

Goal: Demonstrate an understanding of the identification and management of selected common complications of newborns.

Objectives:

- Describe commonly occurring problems of infants of mothers with diabetes.
- List nursing interventions related to hypoglycemia in infants of mothers with diabetes.
- Identify risk factors for development of early-onset group B streptococcal (GBS) infection and HIV infection.
- Describe common signs and symptoms of early-onset GBS infection.
- Discuss the care of the neonate born to an HIV-positive woman.
- Identify signs and symptoms of in utero drug exposure in the neonate.
- Identify common problems found in extremely low-birth-weight infants.

Exercise 1

  CD-ROM Activity

20 minutes

- Sign in to work at Pacific View Regional Hospital on the Obstetrics Floor for Period of Care 4. (*Note*: If you are already in the virtual hospital from a previous exercise, click on **Leave the Floor** and then on **Restart the Program** to get to the sign-in window.)
- Click on **Chart** and then on **202** for Stacey Crider's chart. (*Remember:* You are not able to visit patients or administer medications during Period of Care 4. You are only able to review patients' records.)
- Click on **History and Physical**.
- Scroll down to History of Present Illness.

1. When was Stacey Crider's gestational diabetes diagnosed?

2. How was Stacey Crider's gestational diabetes managed?

➤ • Click on **Nursing Admission** and scroll to Diagnosis on page 1.

3. What was the status of Stacey Crider's gestational diabetes when she was admitted to the hospital at 27 weeks gestation?

Assume that Stacey Crider has given birth and you are now the nurse caring for her baby. Read the section on infants of mothers with diabetes on pages 773-774 in your textbook.

4. The nurse caring for Stacey Crider's infant must recognize that congenital anomalies in the baby born to a mother with diabetes are most likely caused by which of the following? Select all that apply.

_____ Fluctuations in maternal glucose levels

_____ Episodes of ketoacidosis

_____ Maternal hyperglycemia

_____ Fetal hyperinsulinemia

_____ Inability of maternal insulin to cross the placental barrier

5. Tight glycemic controls for the pregnant woman with diabetes is key to the prevention of

complications. It is recommended that the blood glucose levels are _____ to

_____.

6. The risk for congenital anomalies for the infant born to a mother with insulin-dependent diabetes is:
a. 3% to 5%
b. 5% to 8%
c. 7% to 10%
d. 10% to 13%

7. List four nursing interventions to prevent or manage hypoglycemia in Stacey Crider's baby.

Exercise 2

 CD-ROM Activity

 30 minutes

Gabriela Valenzuela was admitted at 34 weeks gestation with vaginal bleeding and uterine contractions following a motor vehicle accident (MVA). Her labor progressed throughout the day on Wednesday, and vaginal delivery is expected.

- Sign in to work at Pacific View Regional Hospital on the Obstetrics Floor for Period of Care 4. (*Note*: If you are already in the virtual hospital from a previous exercise, click on **Leave the Floor** and then on **Restart the Program** to get to the sign-in window.)
- Click on **MAR**, and then on tab **205** for Gabriela Valenzuela's records. (*Remember:* You are not able to visit patients or administer medications during Period of Care 4. You are only able to review patients' records.)

1. What medication has Gabriela Valenzuela been receiving today for GBS prophylaxis?

 • Click on **Return to Nurses' Station**.
- Click on **Chart** and then on **205**.
- Click on **Nurse's Notes**.
- Scroll to the note for Wednesday 1820.

2. What are the findings of Gabriela Valenzuela's cervical exam at this time?

 Assume that Gabriela Valenzuela does give birth today. Read the section on GBS infection on pages 775 and 784 in your textbook.

3. The mortality rate for the infant infected with early-onset GBS is _____ %.

4. All of the following are risk factors for the development of early-onset GBS infection. Place an X beside the risk factor(s) that you know would apply to Gabriela Valenzuela's baby.

_____ Low birth weight

_____ Preterm birth

_____ Rupture of membranes of more than 18 hours

_____ Maternal fever

_____ Previous infant with GBS infection

_____ Maternal GBS bacteriuria

_____ Multiple gestation

5. Early-onset GBS infection most commonly manifests _____

_____. GBS infection usually results from

_____ transmission from the _____.

6. If you were the nurse caring for Gabriela Valenzuela's baby, what signs/symptoms might you see if the baby developed early-onset GBS?

7. _____ Maternal screening and administration of penicillin have significantly decreased the incidence of neonatal GBS infection. (True/False)

Laura Wilson is a G1 P0 at 37 weeks gestation who is also HIV-positive. She was admitted last night with fever, vomiting, and diarrhea to rule out acute abdomen and pyelonephritis. During the day on Wednesday, Laura Wilson began having mild uterine contractions.

• Click on **Return to Nurses' Station**.
• Click on **Chart** and then on **206**.
• Click on **Physician's Notes**.
• Review the note for Wednesday at 0830.

8. Below, record Laura Wilson's HIV-related lab values.

CD4 count

HIV-1 RNA count

➡ • Click on **Physician's Orders**.
   • Scroll to the admission orders for Tuesday at 2130.

9. What is Laura Wilson's current antiretroviral drug regimen?

➡ • Click on **Nurse's Notes**.
   • Scroll down to the note for Wednesday 1830.

10. What event occurred at 1815?

11. Is Laura Wilson in labor at this time? Support your answer.

Laura Wilson is transferred to the Labor and Delivery Unit to give birth. Assume that she does give birth today.

12. All of the following factors, if present, would increase the risk for transmission of HIV to Laura Wilson's baby during the birth process. Place an X beside the risk factor that Laura Wilson has at this time.

_____ High viral load

_____ Low maternal CD4 T-lymphocyte count

_____ Chorioamnionitis

_____ Rupture of membranes more than 4 hours prior to birth

_____ Preterm gestation

13. Give a rationale for your answer to the preceding question.

14. All infants born to HIV-positive mothers should be assumed to be _____.

Diagnosis of HIV infection in the neonate is complicated by _____

_____. The most accurate diagnostic test for newborns

and infants younger than 18 months of age is the _____ assay. Follow-up testing for infants born to HIV-positive mothers is recommended at several

intervals within _____.

15. _____ Currently, neonates born to HIV-positive mothers are treated only with zidovudine to decrease their risk for acquiring the virus. (True/False)

16. Assume that you are the nurse caring for Laura Wilson's baby in the newborn nursery. List several nursing interventions to decrease the risk for viral transmission to the baby.

Exercise 3

 CD-ROM Activity

 30 minutes

In addition to being HIV-positive, Laura Wilson also has a past and current history of substance abuse.

- Sign in to work at Pacific View Regional Hospital on the Obstetrics Floor for Period of Care 4. (*Note:* If you are already in the virtual hospital from a previous exercise, click on **Leave the Floor** and then on **Restart the Program** to get to the sign-in window.)
- Click on **Chart** and then on **206** for Laura Wilson's chart. (*Remember:* You are not able to visit patients or administer medications during Period of Care 4. You are only able to review patients' records.)
- Click on **Nursing Admission**.

1. Complete the chart below with information on Laura Wilson's current use of alcohol and recreational drugs (*Hint:* See page 4 of the Nursing Admission.)

Substance	Reported Use
Alcohol	
Marijuana	
Crack cocaine	

2. Listed below and on the next page are problems often seen in infants exposed prenatally to alcohol, marijuana, or cocaine. Indicate the substance(s) thought to be associated with each problem by marking an X in the proper column(s). (*Note:* More than one drug may be associated with each problem.)

Problem	Alcohol	Marijuana	Cocaine
Craniofacial abnormalities			
Decreased birth weight			
Hyperactivity			
Congenital anomalies			
Developmental delays			
Hypersensitivity to noise and external stimuli			
Difficulty consoling			

3. Fetal alcohol syndrome (FAS) is based on minimal criteria of signs in each of three

   categories: _____,

   _____, and _____. A baby with

   _____ has been
   affected by prenatal exposure to alcohol but does not meet the criteria for FAS.

4. List several interventions to enhance the mother-child relationship that could be used by the
   nurse assigned to work with Laura Wilson and her newborn.

Exercise 4

 CD-ROM Activity

 20 minutes

Kelly Brady was admitted with severe preeclampsia at 26 weeks gestation. Because of her
worsening maternal condition, her baby is delivered by cesarean section on Wednesday.

- Sign in to work at Pacific View Regional Hospital on the Obstetrics Floor for Period of
  Care 4. (*Note*: If you are already in the virtual hospital from a previous exercise, click on
  Leave the Floor and then on **Restart the Program** to get to the sign-in window.)
- Click on **Chart** and then on **203** for Kelly Brady's chart. (*Remember:* You are not able to visit
  patients or administer medications during Period of Care 4. You are only able to review
  patients' records.)
- Click on **Diagnostic Reports**.

1. According to the ultrasound done on Tuesday, what is Kelly Brady's baby's estimated fetal
   weight?

→ • Click on **Consultations**.
- Review the Neonatology Consult for Wednesday at 0800.

2. List common problems for babies born at 26 weeks gestation at Pacific View Regional Hospital, according to the neonatologist who met with Kelly Brady and her husband.

3. If Kelly Brady's baby's actual birth weight is close to her estimated weight, in which weight category will she be placed? Why?

4. Many body systems or functions are likely to be impaired in extremely low birth weight (ELBW) infants. Place an X next to the systems or functions that were also addressed by the neonatologist in his consultation with Kelly Brady. Select all that apply.

_____ Respiratory function

_____ Cardiovascular function

_____ Maintenance of body temperature

_____ CNS function

_____ Maintenance of adequate nutrition

_____ Maintenance of renal function

_____ Maintenance of hematologic status

_____ Resistance to infection

5. List several psychological tasks that Kelly Brady and/or her husband must accomplish as parents.

6. Write a nursing diagnosis appropriate for the Bradys as parents of a premature baby who will have an extended NICU stay.

7. List several nursing interventions to assist the Bradys in accomplishing the parenting tasks you listed in question 5.

Grieving the Loss of a Newborn

 Reading Assignment: The Newborn at Risk (Chapter 24)

Patient: Maggie Gardner, Room 204

Goal: Demonstrate an understanding of the grieving process and how it relates to coping with a current pregnancy.

Objectives:

- Identify the various types of losses as they relate to a pregnancy.
- Describe the stages and phases of the grieving process.
- Identify various methods of coping exhibited by patients who have experienced the loss of a newborn.

Exercise 1

 Writing Activity

15 minutes

Review pages 801-809 in the textbook.

1. Patients may grieve not only the death of a newborn, but also a baby who is born with a

   _____ or _____.

2. List other times that couples may grieve the loss of a newborn.

3. What type of effects do women experience if a pregnancy ends early as a result of miscarriage?

4. Grief involves _____ and

   _____ responses to a major loss.

5. _____ All women and men who undergo a loss receive adequate support. (True/False)

Exercise 2

 CD-ROM Activity

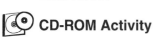 15 minutes

- Sign in to work at Pacific View Regional Hospital on the Obstetrics Floor for Period of Care 4. (*Note*: If you are already in the virtual hospital from a previous exercise, click on **Leave the Floor** and then on **Restart the Program** to get to the sign-in window.)
- From the Nurses' Station, click on **Chart**. (*Remember:* You are not able to visit patients or administer medications during Period of Care 4. You are only able to review patients' records.)
- Click on **204** to open Maggie Gardner's chart.
- Review the **History and Physical**.

  1. How many losses related to pregnancy has Maggie Gardner experienced?

- Click on the **Nursing Admission**.

  2. According to the Nursing Admission, what is the first piece of evidence that Maggie Gardner's previous losses are affecting her current pregnancy and care? (*Hint*: Review the first five sections.)

• Click on the **Consultations** tab.
 • Scroll down to review the Pastoral Consult.

3. To what does Maggie Gardner attribute her inability to have a child?

4. List three therapeutic measures that the chaplain can use to assist Maggie Gardner through these feelings as part of her grieving process.

5. What did the chaplain accomplish during his time with Maggie Gardner?

Exercise 3

 CD-ROM Activity

 20 minutes

1. What is grief?

2. What are the four tasks of grief?

3. What are the three phases of grief?

4. Mothers are the focus during the loss of an infant; however, the _____

   shares the _____ level of grief.

5. What response typically emerges during intense grief? Why?

6. List three other emotions that are experienced during the phase of intense grief.

7. During the phase of reorganization, what is the most common question asked by the grieving person? Explain.

 • Sign in to work at Pacific View Regional Hospital on the Obstetrics Floor for Period of Care 4. (*Note:* If you are already in the virtual hospital from a previous exercise, click on **Leave the Floor** and then on **Restart the Program** to get to the sign-in window.)

• From the Nurses' Station, click on **Chart** and then on **204** to open Maggie Gardner's chart. (*Remember:* You are not able to visit patients or administer medications during Period of Care 4. You are only able to review patients' records.)

• Click on and review the **History and Physical**.

8. Consider how Maggie Gardner's obstetric history and her current feelings compare with what you have read in your textbook about the reorganization phase of grief. What correlation do you see?

 • Click on **Consultations**.

• Once again scroll down and review the Pastoral Consult, specifically the section titled Effects of Illness on Spirituality.

9. Culture and religion play very large roles in how individuals handle a loss. How has Maggie Gardner handled her losses?